Fibromyalgia

A Handbook
for
Self Care & Treatment

Janet A. Hulme, M.A., P.T.

Fibromyalgia, A Handbook for Self Care & Treatment

First Edition Copyright ©1995 by Phoenix Publishing Co.
Second Edition Copyright © 1997 by Phoenix Publishing Co.

ISBN Number: 0-9644848-4-6

Design & Layout
Meerkat Graphics
Lolo, Montana

Published in the U.S.A. by
Phoenix Publishing Co.
P.O. Box 8231
Missoula, Montana 59807

ACKNOWLEDGEMENTS

Many thanks to Erika Hulme, Abigail Hulme and Richard Hulme for writing and editing portions of this book, to Catherine Goodman, P.T., Maureen Fleming, Ph.D., and Don Nevin, M.D. for encouragement and editing, to Roberta Walsh for editing the second edition, to Peggy Schlesinger, M.D. for inspiring my practice in fibromyalgia, and to all my patients for providing essential information about what works and more importantly what doesn't.

This book is not engaged in medical, psychological, financial, legal or other professional services. The services of competent professionals are recommended for expert assistance.

Other publications
by the author

Beyond Kegels
Fabulous four exercises and more...
to prevent and treat incontinence

FOREWORD

Fifteen years ago, the generalized muscle aches, stiffness and fatigue of fibromyalgia was not usually considered a diagnosis with an accepted treatment protocol by health professionals. Fibromyalgia Syndrome (FMS) was often misdiagnosed as an orthopedic or psychiatric problem with treatment protocols based on those diagnoses.

In 1988 after a career in physical therapy education I started a private practice concentrating on women's health, including fibromyalgia. In conjunction with Peggy Schlesinger, M.D., a rheumatologist, treatment protocols were developed and a support group started for individuals with fibromyalgia in my community. During this same period my two daughters were diagnosed with FMS so I became even more interested in treatment approaches and outcomes.

My experience in the clinic working with clients and at home living with my two daughters has been that individuals with fibromyalgia tolerate the symptoms and unconsciously adapt their daily lives, sometimes in very unproductive ways. This can result in a more and more isolated world with less physical activity, friends, and fun. Deconditioning has been thought to cause fibromyalgia in the past. In fact, it is the other way around in most cases. These individuals were highly active and motivated until fatigue and pain were the reward for physical activity and fun in their lives. Just as a rat who is shocked whenever it tries to eat food eventually quits eating, the individual with fibromyalgia eventually quits being active in the attempt to have more energy and less pain. When this occurs in childhood the effects are even more pronounced.

Since there is yet to be a medication or other treatment that cures fibromyalgia, the emphasis of my work has been to combine self care and management strategies with medical intervention to accomplish the most positive outcome for each individual. The purpose of this book is to provide information to health professionals and individuals with fibromyalgia about the unique combination of medical treatment and self care management. Since it is a chronic condition without a cure it requires that the individual take responsibility for managing his/her own care, accept appropriate care from health professionals, and have the wisdom to know when each is necessary.

The successes of modern medicine have led to the expectation that every problem has a "magic" cure. Some individuals with fibromyalgia have found a medical intervention that relieves their symptoms, but more often the same therapy does not work for others and many times it will not even work for the given individual over the long term. That is why education and self care are so important. FMS individuals must know the choices available to them. Health care professionals need to be knowledgeable about appropriate treatment options for fibromyalgia and be able to offer these options in the order of best expected outcomes.

This book is designed to be read in sections or from cover to cover. If there is a special interest, turn to the chapter that addresses that area. Share the ideas with others who need and want to know more about fibromyalgia.

TABLE OF CONTENTS

PART I – WHAT IS IT? DO I HAVE IT?

CHAPTER ONE

WHAT ARE THE SYMPTOMS?

Janet A. Hulme, P.T.

WHAT IS IT?

Fibromyalgia, fibrositis, and fibromyositis are used to describe the same condition. Fibrositis literally means inflammation of the fibrous connective tissue: this is now known to be untrue, but the term fibrositis has persisted. Myalgia means muscle pain so fibromyalgia would literally mean pain as opposed to inflammation of the soft tissue. Fibromyalgia is now the more accepted term.

It is considered a syndrome and not a disease. Pain is the major complaint and is described by some as a migraine headache of the muscles. Fibromyalgia Syndrome (FMS) is characterized by diffuse pain or tender points present in many muscle groups including the neck, face, back, arms, legs, hands and feet. FMS individuals complain of fatigue and exhaustion and of not feeling rested after a night's sleep. Other complaints include lack of sexual desire and loss of a feeling of well being. Myofascial pain syndrome is sometimes confused with fibromyalgia. Fibromyalgia is systemic while myofascial pain syndrome is a localized phenomena. Fibromyalgia has characteristic tender points, localized areas that are painful when pressure is applied. Myofascial pain syndrome has characteristic trigger points that are painful and also refer pain to other areas when pressure is applied.

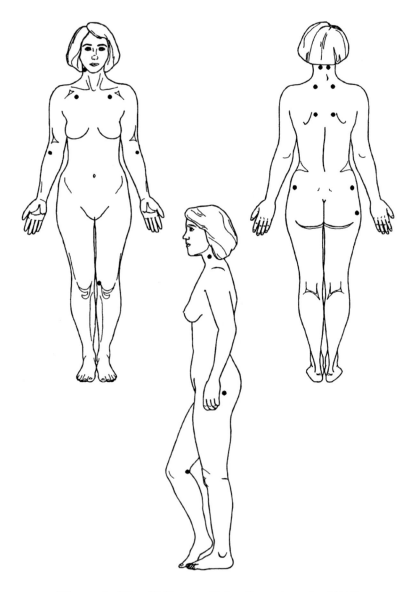

Figure 1: The 18 Tender Point Locations for FMS

Fibromyalgia is described as widespread pain of more than three months' duration in combination with tenderness at specific sites throughout the body. These sites are illustrated in Figure 1.

Tenderness to pressure or touch can vary from a grimace or flinch to intolerable pain. Pain and tenderness are described on both sides of the body, with pain above and below the waist, usually involving the back, neck, chest, arms and legs.

A biofeedback specialist can often demonstrate physiological components of the pain, stiffness, and fatigue of FMS with the use of surface electromyography and thermography. Blood circulation to muscles of the back, arms, legs, hands and feet can be significantly decreased at rest. In some FMS individuals there is noticeable circulation decrease with barometric pressure changes. During exercise, when circulation should normally increase to muscles and the brain, in FMS just the opposite happens and circulation often decreases significantly. Transport of oxygen and food products to muscle cells and removal of waste products is compromised.

The diaphragm, the major breathing muscle, is significantly affected in FMS to the point that it can cease to function as the major breathing muscle and accessory muscles of the neck and upper chest take over. The neck and chest muscles therefore overwork and tender points and/or tightness results.

The resting level of muscle activity during standing and sitting, even reclining, is like the idle on a car engine and can be high or low. In an individual with FMS the muscles' resting level is generally high, the engine is on high idle all the time, which means that even at rest the muscles need more oxygen and food products and accumulate more waste products than normal.

During daily activities such as cleaning, cooking, typing,

and even socializing the muscles used for these activities "overdo" or are at a higher level of activity than muscles of an individual without FMS doing the same tasks. Instead of floating through the activity or social situation the FMS individual's muscles tend to act like "a bull in a china closet" moving fast, strong, and not always in the right direction with the result that the work gets done fast and often well, but the fallout is fatigue and pain on the part of the FMS individual. When the activity is over and the FMS individual is attempting to "rest," those same muscles continue to repeat the activity over and over again even though nothing outwardly is moving, i.e. the muscle activity is in the same pattern as during the activity but at a somewhat decreased level while the individual thinks he/she is resting "quietly." For example, the forearm muscles of any individual writing for several minutes will be highly active in a particular pattern. At completion of writing (hands resting in lap) a non-FMS forearm muscle group activity pattern would be quiet with little activity. The FMS muscle pattern with hands in lap would mimic the writing pattern but at a somewhat decreased amplitude even though the arms appeared to be still. No wonder there is pain and aching for one to two days after a seemingly simple light activity. Those muscles kept doing the activity long after the conscious mind was on to some other task.

The activity of the FMS individual's heart, stomach, intestines, blood vessels and sweat glands, during daily stressors tend to be excessive. These organs over activate resulting in the heart beating faster, the stomach contracting erratically, the smooth muscle of the intestines and bowel contracting abnormally, the breathing rate becoming erratic and rapid, and blood vessels constricting, decreasing blood flow to body parts at times. All these changes occur in response to a relatively mild life stressor. The FMS individual feels heart palpitations, shortness of breath, chest pains, coldness, sweating, numbness, tingling, even panic and anxiety that continues long after the event is over. These responses may linger even after cognitive memory of the initiating event is gone. Cellular memory, a previously suspected but now documented phenomena, may explain this.

Non-FMS individuals experience these changes but the body responses occur in smaller amplitude and for a shorter period of time. The non-FMS responses might include breathing fast, feeling hot or cold, and feeling the heart beating for a few minutes to half an hour, but this is quickly followed by a return to normal. The FMS nervous system's subtleness of response is fragile with both the responses being more exaggerated and the return to a normal state taking more time.

CLINICAL SIGNS AND SYMPTOMS

FMS is sometimes described as the "irritable everything" syndrome. Instead of quieting or inhibiting sensations the FMS individual's nervous system magnifies sensory input. Sounds, light, touch, pressure, smell, taste, heat/cold, and pain can all be exaggerated by the FMS nervous system (Figure 2). Symptoms can be evident throughout the body, but some individuals will feel them in one area more than another (Figure 3). Some periods of time there will be more symptoms, other times very few. Areas of focus (and the average incidence of each) include:

1. Mental and physical fatigue 85%

This is overwhelming tiredness with great effort or inability to move through physical tasks. It can occur with or without precipitating events. Individuals describe mental fatigue, confusion, inability to problem solve or remember even simple tasks.

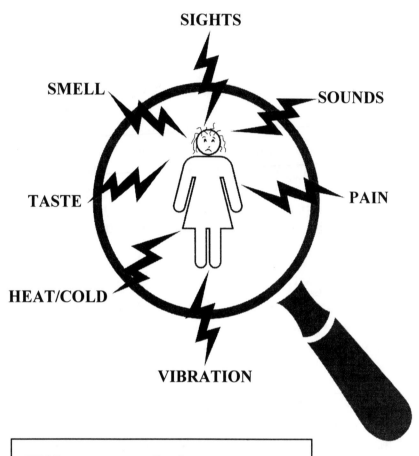

Fibromyalgia
Nervous System
Magnifies Sensations

© J Hulme 1996

Figure 2

6

2. Sleep disturbance / morning fatigue 80%

Deep sleep or delta sleep is when body cells repair and replace themselves and essential hormones for growth and metabolism are released. Growth hormone in an FMS individual is produced in the greatest quantities in the early morning compared to a non-FMS individual who produces it throughout the night, so an FMS individual describes getting his/her best sleep in the morning when others are getting up. Eighty percent of growth hormone is released during deep sleep and growth hormone is essential for normal muscle metabolism and tissue repair. FMS individuals have significantly disrupted deep or Stage 4 sleep. It may take 1-2 hours to get to sleep. Any noise, smell, or other sensory stimuli may lead to arousal. Deep sleep is disrupted by alpha wave sleep, awake-like brain waves that intrude into deep sleep, so it is called alpha-delta sleep anomaly. For others sleep can be disrupted by restless leg syndrome or sleep apnea. The FMS individual sleeps restlessly, waking 2-29 times during the night and wakes feeling stiff, sore, and tired. Muscles maintain a high level of activity at rest, breathing continues shallow and erratic, the circulatory system is often unstable resulting in significantly decreasing body temperature as the night progresses. By contrast, a non-FMS individual usually gets into bed, falls asleep in 15-30 minutes, and sleeps through the night. During the deep sleep muscles go into a deep relaxed state, breathing slows, and circulation maintains a stable body temperature. The individual wakes feeling rested, warm, and relaxed. Feeling tired and sore is not normal!

3. Morning stiffness 75%

This is the persistence of stiffness in the morning for more than 30 minutes. Stiffness can be the feeling of muscles, fascia, or even joints being glued down or jelling when the body is in one position for any period of time.

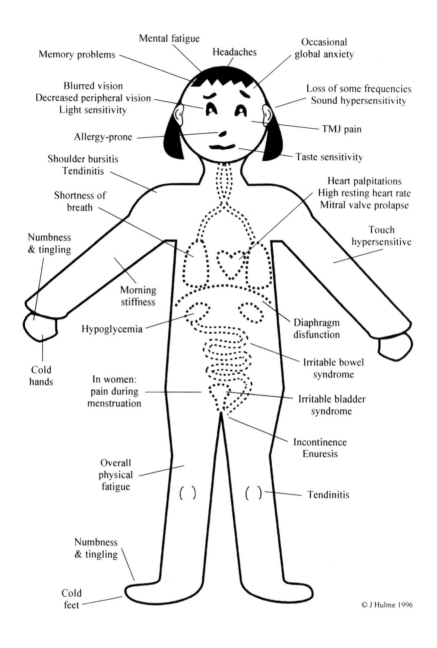

Figure 3: Associated Symptoms of Fibromyalgia

8

4. Global anxiety 72%

Individuals describe a feeling of anxiousness, irritability and overconcern without specific precipitating events. The individual describes a long list of problems – past, present, and potential.

5. Irritable bowel syndrome (IBS) 70%

Specific bowel complaints include alternating diarrhea and constipation, abdominal pain, abdominal gas, and nausea. Gut contractions are normally at 6 cycles/minute. However, in IBS they are at 3 cycles/minute which may give rise to the constipation and abdominal pain, followed by diarrhea.

6. Irritable bladder syndrome, female urethral syndrome 12%

Specific complaints include urinary frequency, as often as every 15-30 minutes, lower abdominal pain and pressure, incontinence (loss of urine), enuresis (night time loss of urine), and interstitial cystitis symptoms (pain and frequency of urination).

7. Headaches 70%

Migraine and tension-type headaches are frequent in FMS individuals. Migraine headaches produce one-sided, throbbing head pain often with associated nausea and hypersensitivity to light and sound. Tension headaches produce a sensation of tightness or pressure across the forehead, on both sides of the head, at the back of the neck, extending into the shoulders. Tension headaches are not necessarily caused by psychological stress or muscle tension.

8. Raynaud's phenomena 38%

Individuals describe cold hands and feet, color changes in tips of fingers and toes.

9. Sicca Syndrome 33%

Individuals describe dry eyes and/or mouth.

10. Depression 20-50%

FMS is not a psychiatric disorder. Depression can occur

in response to pain. Clinical depression is no more prevalent in FMS individuals than in the general population.

11. Paresthesias 50%

Individuals describe numbness and tingling in legs and arms.

12. Subjective Swelling 50%

Individuals describe subjective feeling of swelling, often in hands and feet. It is usually not observable by another person.

13. Pelvic Pain 43%

Recurrent pain in the pelvic area caused by FMS is often misdiagnosed as endometriosis and interstitial cystitis. Dysmenorrhea or painful menstruation is frequent with FMS.

14. Temporomandibular dysfunction (TMD) 25%

TMD causes fascial and head pain with most of the problems related to muscles and ligaments surrounding the jaw joint not necessarily the joint itself.

15. Visual problems up to 95%

Individuals describe blurring, double vision, bouncing images.

16. Auditory problems 31%

At times certain frequencies are difficult for an individual with FMS to hear while at other times hypersensitivity to some frequencies is present.

17. Respiratory dysfunction 33%

Dyspnea or shortness of breath at rest and during physical activity is common. Irregular, erratic breathing patterns are predominant during maximal exertion.

18. Cognitive (memory) problems 71%

Decreased attention span, decreased concentration, and impaired short term memory can have significant implications for learning new behavior and remembering past learning. There may be more time needed to process information and/or increased repetitions to retain a skill.

19. Hypersensitivity to noise, odors, heat or cold 50-60%

There is magnification of environmental stimuli in the FMS individual. Incoming sensations are amplified, sensations from the skin, ears, eyes, nose, and/or mouth are perceived by the individual as excessive (Figure 2).

20. Clumsiness

Suddenly dropping objects, tripping, running into things.

21. Mitral valve prolapse 75%

One of the heart valves bulges more than usual during the heartbeat. It is thought that in most cases the prolapse is caused by an imbalance between the sympathetic and parasympathetic nerve impulses to the heart – termed dysautonomia or dysfunction of the autonomic nervous system.

22. Restless Leg Syndrome (RLS); Periodic Leg Movement Disorder (PLMD) 30-60%

Symptoms described include frequent uncontrolled leg movements, calf muscle cramping, feeling that legs are alive and unable to be still. Numbness, tingling and burning sensations may be present.

23. Allergies

There is frequently a history of hypersensitivity to environmental allergen.

24. Hypoglycemia tendencies 45-50%

Individuals describe weakness, irritability, and disorientation. This may be particularly prevalent after exercise or during the night.

25. Joint Hypermobility 43%

Increased mobility or looseness of joints, for example the thumb can touch the forearm and the elbow hyperextends.

26. Vasopressor Syncope (VDS)

Fainting, light headedness, low blood pressure, and high resting heart rate are typical symptoms. The abnormal heart rate and blood pressure are caused by dysfunctional communication signals from the nervous and hormonal systems.

CHAPTER 2

How Is It Diagnosed? Who Has It?

Janet A. Hulme, P.T.

Fibromyalgia is often diagnosed using the 1990 American College of Rheumatology criteria of:

1. Widespread pain of at least three months' duration.

2. Pain to palpation at a minimum of 11 of the 18 tender point locations. (Tender points are areas of the body that are hypersensitive to pressure or touch.) Tender points are painful and the FMS individual may flinch or unconsciously tighten the area when pressure is applied. In contrast, trigger points are hypersensitive areas of the body that, when pressure is applied, refer pain to a more distant body part as well as being painful over the site. These are present in myofascial pain syndrome.

3. Associated symptoms often are present and include the twenty-six symptoms discussed previously.

4. A normal laboratory profile including complete blood count (CBC), sedimentation rate, antinuclear antibody, rheumatoid factor (RA), muscle enzymes, and thyroid function tests.

CBC measures levels of red, white and platelet cell

numbers. Red blood cells store iron and if red blood cell numbers are decreased fatigue is a symptom. White blood cells fight infection. If they are decreased in number the immune system is impaired. Sedimentation rate (ESR) is the distance the blood cells fall in a test tube in one hour. With infection or inflammation they fall faster. Muscle enzyme tests eliminate the possibility of muscle diseases like muscular dystrophy. Thyroid function test indicates under or overactive thyroid function. Underactive thyroid results in stiff and sore muscles and coldness. If RA factor is positive it indicates rheumatoid arthritis as a possible diagnosis. ANA (Antinuclear Antibodies) tests for autoimmune diseases such as lupus erythematosus. It is a measure of the number of antibodies in the blood.

The blood tests are useful in ruling out areas of misdiagnosis (even though they may accompany fibromyalgia as an additional diagnosis.) Misdiagnoses include:

1. Lyme disease
2. Reaction to silicone implants
3. Polymyalgia rheumatica
4. Rheumatoid arthritis
5. Lupus erythematosus
6. Hypothyroidism
7. Parkinsonism
8. Inflammatory muscle diseases
9. Giant cell arteritis
10. Tendinitis
11. Yeast infections
12. Kawasaki's disease

WHO HAS FIBROMYALGIA?

Approximately 1% of females between 20 and 30 have FMS. Up to 8% of individuals 70 and older experience FMS. There is a female to male ratio of eight or nine to two. The average age at the time of diagnosis is 49 but individuals describe having had symptoms for five or more years before diagnosis. The age range at diagnosis is six to 85 years old. Twenty five percent have a childhood onset, seventy-five percent have adult onset. The onset is often insidious. Twenty percent of FMS occurs rapidly after surgery or trauma. Approximately five to ten percent occurs following a febrile, usually a viral, illness. Twenty-five percent of FMS individuals have one or more other medical problems, i.e. degenerative joint disease, inflammatory arthritis, tendinitis, clinical depression, lupus erythematosus, or thyroid disease.

Even though FMS is described primarily in adults, children experience the same symptoms but are often undiagnosed or misdiagnosed. There is some indication that up to eight percent of the school population exhibit FMS symptoms. It is classified as juvenile primary fibromyalgia syndrome (JPFS). The criteria are:

1. Presence of diffuse musculoskeletal aches, pains and stiffness for at least 3 months.

2. Presence of a least ten typical and discrete tender points.

3. Symptoms modulated by such factors as weather, physical activity and anxiety/stress.

4. Non-restorative sleep.

5. Absence of arthritic, inflammatory, endocrine or infectious processes.

6. Normal standard laboratory tests.

Children complain of diffuse pain, stiffness, feeling of swelling, fatigue, poor sleep, waking tired, headaches, numbness/tingling, and anxiety.

CHAPTER 3

WHAT CAUSES FIBROMYALGIA?

Janet A. Hulme, P.T.

The cause of fibromyalgia is unknown at this time. The communication system of the body and mind, i.e. the nerves and chemicals (hormones) that send messages between organs and other body tissue (muscles), and the brain functions abnormally giving too much information sometimes and not enough at other times. Recent research findings indicate that FMS runs in families and there may be a genetic predisposition to the dysfunction of the communication network (possibly on human chromosome 6). The genetic predisposition to the communication dysfunction alone can cause FMS. However, in some FMS individuals the communication dysfunction seems to be triggered by physical trauma such as a motor vehicle accident; repetitive motion such as work on an assembly line or using a computer repetitively; emotional trauma such as a death or divorce; environmental stress such as excessive noise, vibration, light or temperature. In some individuals a flu-like illness preceded the fibromyalgia symptoms.

As I. Jon Russell describes it, "something (is) wrong in the central nervous system that processes a person's ability to perceive pain." We know that Substance P (SP), a neurotransmitter for pain, is elevated in FMS individuals to nearly three times that of non-FMS individuals. Pain inhibition neurotransmitters include serotonin, norepinephrine, GABA, and enkephalins. Decreased cerebral spinal fluid levels of serotonin, norepinephrine and dopamine have been reported in FMS individuals. Decreased serotonin can lead to symptoms including pain, fatigue, mitral valve prolapse, sinus congestion, night sweats, anxiety, and compulsivity.

A disturbance in the limbic system function has been described. The limbic system includes the hypothalamus and the pituitary glands and functions to regulate fatigue, pain, sleep, weight, appetite, libido, respiration, temperature, blood pressure, memory, attention, concept formation, mood, vigilance, immune and endocrine systems, and the modulation of the autonomic nervous system. The hypothalamus produces chemical messengers that signal the pituitary gland to release hormones that act on specific organs to regulate body functions. Studies have shown decreased hormonal output within this system. Both growth hormone and cortisol production appear low in FMS. Impaired cell repair and growth and fatigue are just two of the results of decreased cortisol and growth hormone. To complete the feedback loop norepinephrine, dopamine, and serotonin are thought to stimulate the production of growth hormone by the pituitary gland.

Cerebral blood flow, determined by SPECT scan imaging, is often abnormal in FMS individuals. A marked reduction in blood flow has been found in both hemispheres but it is greater in the right hemisphere's temporal and frontal lobes in FMS patients with widespread pain. The thalamus and caudate nuclei region exhibit decreased blood flow in FMS individuals and are associated with low pain thresholds. This region has connections to the limbic system and is thought to be involved in memory/concentration tasks and pain regulation.

Blood flow to arm and legs, particularly hands and feet, can be significantly decreased in FMS. The fight or flight, sympathetic portion of the autonomic nervous system causes constriction of the blood vessels which can lead to cold hands and feet. An FMS individual describes being core cold at times, or feeling alternately hot and cold. Night sweats are common. Coldness can sometimes be a predictive symptom for increased pain and fatigue. Interrupting the constriction of blood vessels can prevent the chain reaction of decreased circulation, increased pain and fatigue symptoms.

CHAPTER 4

DOES THIS PICTURE OF FIBROMYALGIA FIT ME?

Ellen S. Silverglat, M.S.W.
Erika Hulme
Janet A. Hulme, P.T.

Four individuals with fibromyalgia agreed to tell their unique stories. Each one experienced symptoms in his/her own way yet there is a similar thread throughout.

FIBROMYALGIA AND ME, ADOLESCENT ONSET

My story of fibromyalgia is one of pain and confusion, as well as understanding, coping and solutions. I was diagnosed with fibromyalgia as a freshman in high school, but the pain preceded the diagnosis by many years. In fact, I cannot remember a time when I haven't had pain and headaches that often severely limited me.

My memories preceding my diagnosis are of confusion, loneliness and misunderstanding. I remember feeling confused about my pain because no one understood it or could figure out why I was in pain. I doubted my own feelings and often thought that maybe I was imagining it, that it wasn't real. I felt like a hypochondriac. Because of the pain and the confusion I never wanted to go out and play or be physically active. Instead, I read a lot and stayed in my room. Sometimes the only place I felt safe and comfortable was in my room and I would hide out there for hours. I felt out of place with other kids my age because all of them wanted to play sports and games that I wasn't interested in. I felt a push from everyone to do things out of doors and sometimes this would turn to anger when I wouldn't participate in the activities.

One of the hardest things for me was not knowing what was the matter. A part of me wanted to be out with my friends, just like a "normal" kid. Yet, I was always so tired and achy that I felt like I couldn't do anything. That part of me kept me down and there was always this conflict of interest.

I went to doctor after doctor for specific problems that I would later learn all stemmed from the fibromyalgia. I went to a specialist for knee pain and my family practitioner for stomach pain several times. Nothing was ever completely explained. The final event that led to a diagnosis was shoulder pain that prevented me from lifting my arm over my head. A rheumatologist finally diagnosed my fibromyalgia in the spring of '89, at the end of my freshman year in high school.

Of course, the pain did not disappear following the diagnosis. Knowing what I had was still just the first step in understanding and coping with the pain I had been experiencing. In high school there were two periods of time when I felt so bad that I didn't go to school for days at a time. My stomach always hurt and I felt like all I could do was lie in bed and sleep. I guess I was kind of depressed, but at the time I wouldn't have described it that way. It was more just an exhaustion dragging me down and making me not want to get out of bed. Both times I only got better with a lot of encouragement from my mother. She made me get out of bed and do some walking and other daily activities that I would have neglected. Finally, I would start to feel better and slowly get back into my old life and activities.

There have been many obstacles to overcome in living with fibromyalgia. One of the toughest has been dealing with people. It is really difficult explaining to friends what is the matter with me and how it limits my life. I can't just say "I broke my arm" or "I have mono." People understand those limitations and can respond to them. Fibromyalgia requires much more explaining and I don't even totally understand it, so how do I try to explain something I don't comprehend? Family members come to understand enough to get by, but even they don't really know what it is like or how it affects everything I do.

Friends are harder to deal with. They want you to be fun and active with them all the time. It has been even harder with my teachers. Usually I don't even try to explain it to them because when I have tried I have gotten blank stares. They say they understand and then it is pushed into the recesses of their minds or completely forgotten.

I've been on and off different medications since my diagnosis. I've found that I am sensitive to most medication so a majority of the time I cope with the pain without medication. I took one medication for a little over half a year until I had an adverse reaction to it. It lowered my blood pressure and raised my heart rate causing dizziness and faintness. I then tried another medication, but had a terrible reaction that caused cold sores and a skin rash.

The thing I hate most is the limits that fibromyalgia places on my life. I always have to think before I participate in any activity that I know might end up making me miserable the next day. The repercussions my actions might have on my body always have to be a major concern. The hardest thing for me is putting myself first, no matter what I have to put aside to do it, even if it is studying for an exam or not going out with friends. I have found that if I am the priority I can do more and the pain actually interferes less with my life. I still go out and have fun with my friends, and still get good grades. I just have to plan better and make the most of the times that I feel good.

It has taken a long time to acknowledge and respond quickly to the clues my body gives me that help me deal with this on a daily basis. I've learned that if I am feeling grouchy or feel myself getting annoyed easily with everything I need to think about what is really bothering me. Usually it is a headache and I now know that I need to lie down and relax to help it go away. To help care for myself I take a little time each day by myself to just relax and not think about anything. This time helps me to focus on quiet and calm. I also try to have fun each day, no matter how much I have to do.

It goes without saying that growing up with fibromyalgia has affected my life. I can look back and see that the reason I stayed inside and read rather than playing games with my friends was probably because I was hurting or had a headache. In some ways I think I missed out on a lot, but I am also a stronger person. I am much more aware of my limits and abilities.

Right now I am a senior in college. Some days are bad, but for the most part I feel good and am able to be a successful student. I know that I am very fortunate to be doing as well as I am and that I am able to lead what is for the most part a normal life. It isn't easy, but I manage. I think that is the key word for people with fibromyalgia, MANAGEMENT.

A WOMAN'S STORY

I have been asked to share my story about living with fibromyalgia. Boy that sounds dramatic to me, because I don't think I live differently than anyone else . . . denial?

most likely. Let me tell you a little about myself. I am almost 30 years old. I grew up in Europe, was raised by successful and supportive parents. My mom never ran out of energy, but I do remember her being in pain . . . and she still is. I am the oldest of three children. As a young child I was very physically active but I often complained of pain. I think my mom thought I was "getting hurt" and suggested I start swimming. What a great idea! I love to swim. I swam competitively in high school and college and was ranked at a national and international level.

I now know that I have fibromyalgia. I had to be very persistent with my doctors to have them look at fibromyalgia as the possible cause of my problems. I complained of some part of my body aching or hurting every day and swallowed up to 20 Advil a day. I didn't realize other people didn't hurt like this. I had chest pain and shortness of breath. I experienced vision problems but the glasses they prescribed did not help. I felt fatigued a lot. The physician said it was normal to be tired with all the swimming I did, but none of my friends were as worn down as I was and some even swam longer distances. I had "tendinitis" of every tendon possible which was treated with ice (which I hated) and anti-inflammatory drugs. The things I never complained of because I didn't want to be labeled as crazy included: transient concentration problems, inability to eat certain foods, irritability, mood swings, extreme abdominal pains, bowel problems, inability to cope with noises and inability to be rational when I was tired. Associated with the fibromyalgia, I had heart problems diagnosed as idiopathic arrhythmia in 1993. Initially I was unable to climb a flight of stairs without multiple rests. I was experiencing angina just sitting around. Eventually I found a cardiologist who worked with me and encouraged my athletics again.

Today I am the director of physical therapy at a major

urban hospital. I am also enrolled in an MBA program on a part-time basis and guest lecture at a local physical therapy school. I compete in master's swimming and in triathlons. To do this I must take care of myself in very specific ways. I avoid extreme temperature changes. I have to acclimate to altitude slowly. I avoid extreme emotional situations and stresses when possible. I prevent hypoglycemic attacks by eating frequent and regular small meals. I have to get 8-10 hours sleep a night. I take medication and vitamins regularly. I avoid caffeine and drink plenty of liquid. I accept my fatigue days and limit my activities on those days.

It is wonderful to have many good days and to be able to effectively treat the bad days. My husband is a big reason for me to finally get the proper care. He laughs with me when I tell him my hair hurts. I know that getting frustrated and angry only makes me worse (that doesn't mean I don't get frustrated and angry at times). I feel healthy. I still have big dreams. My biggest dream is to finish the Iron Man Triathlon in Hawaii. Some people would say that my "plate" is full. Yes, it is and I don't know it to be different.

A SECOND WOMAN'S STORY

About five years ago I noticed a tremor in my left hand and that my fingertips were turning white at times. Then my leg muscles started twitching, sometimes making my whole leg move, especially at night. I felt very tired and I had periodic diarrhea so I thought I had the flu but it never went away. Over several months the tremors in my arms and legs became less but the aching in my neck and back was so much that I couldn't sit at my desk and work for more than two hours, and that exhausted me for the rest of the day. I quit my job four years ago and have not been able to work since then.

There are some days now when I get up, take my shower,

get dressed and do some light housework before noon. After doing this I have to rest for at least two hours in the afternoon so I have enough energy to fix something easy for dinner by 5:00 p.m. Then at night I watch TV or play cards with my husband, but it even hurts to hold the cards in my hands some nights. On bad days I am in bed most of the day because I hurt and have no energy.

I have been to at least a dozen different doctors and tried every medication in the book, but I have severe side effects to most of the ones I've tried and the others haven't helped. I am better than I was four years ago and I plan to start a typing service in my home so I can work at my own pace. I have always liked to work and just one or two hours a day will be better than nothing.

A MAN'S STORY

I am a construction worker and injured my right shoulder two years ago pulling cable. It was diagnosed as a rotator cuff injury. I had physical therapy and finally surgery one year ago. When I went back to work I felt pain in both shoulders and into my back and neck. My right hand started going numb when I drove truck or pulled cable. I have a high tolerance for pain but work tired me out so much that when I got home I was out of sorts and went to bed early.

Even though I went to bed early I woke in the morning feeling terrible. Sometimes I woke up ten times during the night. It took me until noon to work out all the kinks at work. I felt like Frankenstein in the morning, feeling very stiff and moving awkwardly. By afternoon I could bend and reach more easily.

I used to work out in the gym and lap swim 3-4 nights a week after work. I hated to admit it but I was too tired and sore to do it. If I went twice a month I was lucky. My two sons complained that I wouldn't play baseball with them but when I pitched more than a half dozen balls I started to get a headache and my back and shoulder started hurting. My family life had really gone downhill. I slept on the couch half the time because I was so restless and up so many times my wife said she couldn't sleep. I pushed through the pain but my family said they didn't know me anymore and they saw what the pain was doing to me more than I did. I guess I just got used to it and forgot about what it used to be like.

Six months later.

I am doing a lot better now. I started on medication six months ago and also learned some biofeedback and pacing techniques. I had six weeks more physical therapy tailored more for fibromyalgia than a shoulder injury. We do some of the physical therapy at home when I have more pain than usual. I am continuing to work and now I work out 2-3 days a week at the gym and swim or walk the other days. I sleep well most nights and don't feel like a zombie when I wake up. However, I still take a hot shower and loosen up first thing in the morning. My boys say I can throw the ball better and I'm more fun to be around. My wife says I still don't do enough around the house when I get home but she will put up with it to have her husband back.

CHAPTER 5

WHAT CAN PHYSICIANS DO TO HELP?

Peggy R. Schlesinger, M.D.
Muriel R. Friedman, M.D.
Barbara Penner, P.T.
Janet A. Hulme, P. T.

A physician who knows about fibromyalgia is the keystone of the health care team. Most frequently this is an internist, a family practice physician, a physiatrist, or a rheumatologist. The important key is his/her knowledge and interest in treating fibromyalgia and the ability to listen to the patient's needs and priorities.

The physician will take a complete history of present and past problems. He/she will review the results of blood tests and X-rays as well as results of special tests used to eliminate other illnesses which could cause the same symptoms. The physician will perform a physical exam which includes palpation of tender points and assessment of functional movement of neck, back, arms and legs. The diagnosis of fibromyalgia is made from the results of the evaluation.

Once the diagnosis is made, the physician recommends appropriate medications and follows up on the medication's effectiveness and any side effects. The physician coordinates the health care team in developing treatment strategies. Treatment strategies include techniques for pain relief, sleep disturbance relief, daily self care management, self care crisis management, and quality of life restoration which may include a return to work. Fibromyalgia is not a curable problem so the physician's ultimate role is to assist the individual in taking control of his/her life, taking over self care for pain, fatigue and stiffness. The physician assists the individual in knowing when and how the medical team can help.

Some physician specialists become involved with FMS individuals for associated problems. Urologists diagnose and treat bladder problems. Since fibromyalgia affects smooth muscle and circulation in the bladder, symptoms of frequent urination, enuresis (uncontrolled leaking of urine), lower abdominal discomfort and flank or kidney pain in the absence of test findings of infection, obstruction or tumors can often be linked to fibromyalgia. When the symptoms are chronic (1-2 years) and include frequent urination (multiple times an hour during the day and more than two times at night), feeling the urge to urinate but having very little flow, a bloated feeling of discomfort/pain in the lower abdomen, the diagnosis may be interstitial cystitis, fibromyalgia, or a combination of the two. Acute pain in the mid back region without positive findings on IVP, CAT or MRI can be ischemic or muscle pain of fibromyalgia rather than kidney problems. Urethral syndrome symptoms (frequent urination and discomfort with urination) can be caused by fibromyalgia. FMS is usually not the primary cause of incontinence but it can be a significant contributing factor such that until the FMS is treated appropriately the incontinence symptoms will persist at least periodically. Fibromyalgia can be involved in urge, mixed and enuresis types of incontinence much more than stress incontinence (leaking with jumping, running or coughing).

In all the urological disorders mentioned, treatment includes medication and reeducation of the pelvic muscles, bladder, and abdominal muscles via exercise, massage, and physiological quieting.

Abdominal and pelvic pain can be a predominant symptom for some FMS individuals. An obstetrician/ gynecologist and gastroenterologist may be involved in differentiating the symptoms of tumors and infections of the reproductive organs and intestines from fibromyalgia. During pregnancy, the biomechanical and hormonal changes may increase back pain, thoracic outlet syndrome or carpal tunnel symptoms. When the obstetrician is aware the individual has FMS, the care can be specialized to provide for optimum comfort and function. Increased pain symptoms respond well to treatments such as gentle exercise, massage, heat and modalities.

An orthopedic surgeon diagnoses and treats musculoskeletal disorders, problems with bones, joints, and soft tissue (muscle, tendon, capsule). Fibromyalgia can be misdiagnosed as tendinitis when there is pain and tenderness around tendons and joints of the shoulder, elbow, hip, knee, and ankle. It can be misdiagnosed as thoracic outlet syndrome, carpal tunnel syndrome, ulnar nerve compression and even sciatica when there is numbness, tingling and shooting pain that comes and goes. An orthopedic surgeon who is familiar with fibromyalgia will ask the key questions and evaluate to determine if the problem is fibromyalgia or a combination of fibromyalgia and an orthopedic problem. Many FMS individuals give a history of having multiple tendinitis diagnoses over the years. Back pain is prominent in fibromyalgia. A knowledgeable orthopedic surgeon will evaluate appropriately to differentiate disc disease or compression from fibromyalgia since the pain description can be the same in many cases.

A neurologist evaluates and treats dysfunction of the nervous system. Diagnostic tests are performed to eliminate diseases of the nervous system such as multiple sclerosis, Parkinsons disease or amyotrophic lateral sclerosis. A neurologist performs nerve conduction velocity tests to determine if the pain, numbness, and tingling the individual describes is a nerve compression problem such as carpal tunnel syndrome, ulnar nerve compression, or thoracic outlet syndrome.

Where there is another diagnosis in conjunction with fibromyalgia, treating the fibromyalgia first, then seeing what symptoms remain has been the most effective approach. It is advisable that any physician a FMS individual chooses should have a working knowledge of fibromyalgia and its implications.

As one FMS individual said about finding a doctor. "I have looked long and hard for my doctor. The one I have now listens, always gives me options for treatment, involves my family, and encourages me to be independent and try new things. He is wonderful about keeping up on new medications that might help."

CHAPTER 6

What Medications Can Help?

Janet A. Hulme, P.T.
Gayle Cochran, Pharm.D.

Drug treatments will help some individuals and not others. Some medications act immediately while some take weeks or months to have an effect. Some medications become less effective with long term use so a different medication must be tried. At this point in fibromyalgia treatment medications are often used on a trial and error basis to find which ones are most effective to relieve the individual's symptoms and have the fewest side effects. It is important to take the medication over the long term, not just when symptoms are present. Like a diabetic, there is a chemical imbalance or lack of certain chemicals needed for health, and the medication is needed on a regular basis to best maintain symptom relief.

SUMMARY OF SYMPTOM RELIEF MEDICATIONS

ANXIETY – Benzodiazepines

SLEEP DISTURBANCE – Tricyclic antidepressants, Benzodiazepines, Calcium, Melatonin, Valerian

FATIGUE – Selective serotonin reuptake inhibitors (SSRI)

IRRITABLE BOWEL SYNDROME – Antispasmodics (Bentyl, Levsin), Tricyclic antidepressants, Imodium, Magnesium, Vitamin C, Dietary Fiber

IRRITABLE BLADDER SYNDROME – Tricyclic antidepressants, Urised

HEADACHES – Nonsteroidal anti-inflammatories, Calcium channel blockers, Imitrex

RESTLESS LEG SYNDROME – Sinemet, Klonopin, Vitamin E, Calcium and Magnesium combined

DESCRIPTION OF COMMONLY USED MEDICATIONS

TRICYCLIC ANTIDEPRESSANTS (TCA)
Function: Increase CNS neurotransmitter levels
        (serotonin and/or norepinephrine)
Effect: Sedation, diminish fatigue, decrease pain, elevate
        mood
Dose: 5-75 mg often at bedtime – dose varies with drug
Side Effects: Racing heart, nightmares, hangover
        sedation, dry mouth, urinary retention,
        constipation

Examples: amitriptyline (Elavil)
            nortriptyline (Pamelor)
            doxepin (Sinequan)
            desipramine (Norpramin)

CYCLOBENZAPRINE (Flexeril)
A tricyclic amine, it is a muscle relaxant.

NEFAZODONE (Serzone)
Function: Inhibits uptake of serotonin and
            norepinephrine
Effect: Decrease pain, diminish fatigue
Side Effects: Nausea, headaches, postural hypotension
Note: Not to be taken with monoamine oxidase
            inhibitors

NONSTEROIDAL ANTI-INFLAMMATORIES – (NSAIDs)
Function: Inhibits prostaglandin synthesis
Effect: Blocks pain and inflammation at local tissue level
Dose: 600-800 mg/day for analgesic level
Side Effects: Nausea, stomach pain, ulcers, fluid
            retention, renal toxicity in older
            individuals
Examples: ibuprofen (Motrin, Advil)
            naproxen (Naprosyn, Aleve)

BENZODIAZEPINES
Function: Increase GABA (gamma aminobutryric acid)
            which acts on thalamus to inhibit anxiety
Effect: Diminish pain and anxiety, increase sleep
Dose: Varies with particular agent
Side Effects: Sedation, depression
Examples: alprazolam (Xanax)
            clonazepam (Klonopin)
Note: Dependency/addictive qualities

TRAMADOL (Ultram)

Function: Increases serotonin and norepinephrine, increases opioid reception; a synthetic analgesic

Effect: Inhibits pain perception, decreases pain

Dose: 50 mg, 2-4/day

Side Effects: Dizziness, nausea, constipation, headaches, postural hypotension

Note: Dependency/addictive qualities

ZOLPIDEM (Ambien)

Function: Non-benzodiazepine sedative/hypnotic

Effect: Increased duration of sleep, decreased time to get to sleep

Dose: 5-10 mg

Side Effects: Memory problems, daytime drowsiness, dizziness, headache, nausea

Note: Short term treatment of insomnia only, 7-10 days, dependency/addictive qualities

SEROTONIN REUPTAKE INHIBITORS

Function: Blocks destruction of serotonin so its effects last longer (controls food intake, temperature regulation, anxiety)

Effect: Diminish pain, fatigue, and anxiety; improve mood

Dose: 20-200mg depending on agent

Side Effects: Anxiety, nervousness, insomnia, tremor, dizziness

Examples: fluoxetine (Prozac)
sertraline (Zoloft)
paroxetine (Paxil)
venafaxine (Effexor)

CALCIUM CHANNEL BLOCKERS
Function: Dilates arteries, lowers blood pressure, inhibits contraction of smooth vascular muscle, especially of the cerebral arteries

Effect: Decrease pain, headaches, fatigue, memory problems; improves circulation

Dose: Up to 30 mg 2-3 times a day or once daily slow release 60 mg (depends on drug)

Side Effects: Decreased blood pressure, flushing, swelling in feet, constipation, dizziness

Examples: nimodipine (Nimotop) 30 mg
diltiazem 60-240 mg (many strengths and trade names)

VASODILATORS
Function: Vasodilation of arteries or veins

Effect: (Experimental in nature) diminish pain, fatigue, anxiety, memory deficits

Dose: Varies with agent

Side Effects: Light headedness, headaches, tachycardia reflex

Examples: Nitroglycerin 0.4 mg sublingual
Hydralazine 25 mg

ESTROGEN REPLACEMENT THERAPY
Can stabilize hormonal levels in females, may improve cognitive function and improve vasomotor stability.

GROWTH HORMONE
Nutropin: At this time experimental only; release stimulated by serotonin and dopamine.

COMBINATION THERAPIES
1. PROZAC and SINEQUAN
   Restlessness caused by Prozac balanced by Sinequan quieting
2. PROZAC and ELAVIL
   Elavil at night and Prozac in the morning
3. KLONOPIN and SINEQUAN
   Klonopin gets you to sleep, Sinequan keeps you there
4. XANAX and NSAID (Motrin)
   antianxiety, analgesia

Note: Any sedating antidepressant at bedtime may be used with any of the SSRIs in the morning, for example trazadone (Desyrel), a sedative, used with sertraline (Zoloft) an SSRI.

TRIGGER POINT INJECTIONS
Trigger points, when pressure is applied to the area, are painful at the site and refer pain to other areas of the body. They are a sign of a myofascial pain pattern or syndrome. Tender points are exquisitely painful at the site of pressure only and are a sign of fibromyalgia.

Injections into trigger points in FMS are appropriate if there is also myofascial pain in conjunction with FMS symptoms. The trigger points are injected with:
1. Lidocaine, procaine (local anesthetics)
2. Cortisone – in small amounts, less frequently. There may be increased pain for up to 48 hours after the injection, then there should be a decrease in pain over the long term. Systemic side effects almost never occur if the volume injected is below 5 cc, but this is dependent on the potency of the steroid.

ANTIYEAST REGIMENS
1. Lactobacillus Acidophilus
2. Co Enzyme Q
3. Vitamin B 12
4. Fluconazole for 1-3 weeks, Nystatin as maintenance

LOCAL ANESTHETIC SPRAYS / OILS / CREAMS
1. Fluoromethane spray – see Chapter 10
2. Topical creams
    trolamine salicylate 10% (Myoflex)
    capsaicin (Zostrix) cream decreases pain by
        decreasing substance P
3. Essential Oils – see Chapter 10

NUTRITIONAL
1. VITAMIN C 500-3,000 MG
2. VITAMIN Bs 25-50 MG
3. VITAMIN E 200-400 IU
4. MAGNESIUM 500-800 MG
5. CALCIUM 1000-1500 MG
6. MALIC ACID 1200-1400 MG

More details about nutrition are available in Chapter 10.

MEDICATIONS FOR JUVENILE FIBROMYALGIA SYNDROME

These include cyclobenzaprine, amytriptyline, and trazodone. Before adolescence, education and biofeedback are recommended initially and medication is used only if the education and biofeedback is not adequate.

HERBAL / NATURAL PRODUCTS

1. Licorice – Use natural not synthetic form. Used to increase blood volume and decrease low blood pressure in vasopressor syncope.
2. Melatonin – Secreted by pineal gland and made from serotonin. It helps set the sleep/wake cycle.
3. Valerian – Used to treat sleep disturbance.
4. Echinacea – Used to decrease pain.
5. Calms Forte – Used to improve sleep and anxiety.
6. Rhus Toxicodendron – Used to treat stiffness.
7. Ginger – Used to improve irritable bowel syndrome.
8. Cayenne – Used to improve circulation and digestion, to decrease pain.
9. Peppermint – Used to improve digestion and decrease intestinal cramping.
10. Chamomile – Used to improve sleep and decrease intestinal cramping.

CHAPTER 7

WHAT CAN TRADITIONAL AND ALTERNATIVE MEDICINE DO TO HELP?

Gail E. Nevin, P.T.
Janet A. Hulme, P.T.

WHAT CAN PHYSICAL AND OCCUPATIONAL THERAPY DO?

Physical and occupational therapists (P.T./O.T.) are important members of the team approach to managing fibromyalgia. They are helpful in reaching the goals of decreasing pain, fatigue, and sleep disturbance. P.T./O.T. direct management of exercise to reach the goals of optimal fitness while maintaining decreased pain and fatigue, and increasing endurance for daily activities. P.T./O.T. develop strategies for work modification, applying ergonomic techniques to increase efficiency and decrease pain.

PAIN CONTROL

HEAT

Pain control is often the first priority. Heat in the form of hot packs and heating pads, and hot water in the form of hot tubs, hot showers or whirlpools, decreases pain by increasing circulation and relaxing muscle and joint structures. Cold is also used at times for pain control. Crushed ice, cold packs, and ice cups produce numbness and decreased pain. A combination of heat and cold alternating every 5-7 minutes for 20 minutes can be beneficial. Fluoromethane spray and heat is also used to decrease pain.

Ultrasound therapy is helpful at times. High frequency sound waves are transmitted from the head of the equipment to the muscles, ligaments and fasciae through a thin film of conductive gel. Ultrasound waves cause vibration of muscle cells increasing circulation and relaxing muscle tightness. Ultrasound is often effective at .5-.75 watts per centimeter squared, pulsed for 3-5 minutes.

ELECTRICAL MODALITIES

Equipment using electrical current may assist in pain control for fibromyalgia. Equipment that can be helpful includes high voltage galvanic stimulation, interferential current stimulation, and microamperage stimulation. Electrical current in the various forms increases circulation and facilitates muscle relaxation as well as decreasing pain. Electrical stimulation is delivered through moist pads placed over muscle areas which are connected to a piece of equipment via wires. The electric stimulation causes pulsation and a "buzzing" may be felt during the treatment. High voltage galvanic stimulation is often effective at 50-100 volts, 80 pulses per second, negative polarity, 2.5 seconds reciprocal for 20 minutes. Microamperage is often effective at .5 mv for 20 minutes using silver-silver chloride electrodes.

PHYSIOLOGICAL QUIETING

P.T./O.T. assist in developing strategies for the sleep

disturbance prevalent in fibromyalgia. To improve sleep, equipment to eliminate noise, light, smells, and temperature changes is recommended. Physiological quieting audio tapes are often effective for improving deep sleep. See Chapter 10 for an in-depth discussion of physiological quieting.

EXERCISE

As pain, fatigue, and sleep disturbance improve, fitness in strength and endurance becomes a priority. P.T./O.T. develop progressive exercise programs for joint and muscle flexibility, muscle strength, and cardiovascular (heart and lung) fitness. Range of motion and stretching exercises decrease stiffness and improve flexibility. Fluoromethane spray and heat can often increase flexibility while decreasing pain and stiffness (see Chapter 10). Isometric (pushing against an immovable object), isokinetic or isotonic (moving an arm or leg through space) exercise increases muscle strength. Cardiovascular fitness through aerobic exercise means gradually increasing the strength of the heart, lungs, and circulation. Walking, biking, or swimming for 20-30 minutes daily is recommended.

Exercise is often accomplished with less pain and faster progression if done in a warm pool (see Chapter 11). Water at shoulder height significantly decreases the effect of gravity on an individual's body. There is a feeling of weightlessness. A warm pool (85-92°F) increases circulation and improves muscle relaxation. Using a hot tub before and after exercise is also helpful.

Endurance in daily activities improves as strength and flexibility increases. P.T./O.T. tasks include developing daily pacing, energy conservation, work/rest cycles and fun/work cycles in conjunction with the vocational goals of the individual. Altering daily tasks such as dressing, cooking, driving, writing, and telephoning, so that they are efficient and pain free is essential. P.T./O.T. can assist in maintaining job tasks through ergonomic and equipment changes and scheduling modifications.

Over months and years, P.T./O.T. reevaluations provide tracking of the individual's progress so he/she knows there is improvement, that they are doing better even though the steps taken are small and there are setbacks along the way. They provide reinforcement in terms of learning to manage and continuing to try new skills and experiences.

MASSAGE THERAPY

Massage can be helpful for pain relief, improved circulation, relaxation of muscles and removal of waste product build up. Massage needs to start gently, pain is not gain in massage for fibromyalgia. As the muscles release, deeper massage may be appropriate. Special techniques, including craniosacral and myofascial release techniques can be appropriate and beneficial. Massage therapists, physical therapists, occupational therapists, nurses, and chiropractors are all individuals trained in massage.

For self massage, balls, theracane, even the sharp corner of a wall can be used to assist with pressure techniques. Tender point pressure and acupressure, as well as relaxation massage techniques, can be learned by the individual and a supportive family member. Using essential oils with massage may bring additional pain relief.

MANIPULATION THERAPY

Manipulations and adjustments of joints to properly align the vertebra or other body segments can be beneficial in decreasing the pain and muscle tension and increasing circulation and nerve flow for fibromyalgia individuals. Spinal alignment is temporary if muscle tightness and spasm alters vertebral position. Osteopathic physicians, chiropractic physicians, and physical therapists are trained in this area of treatment.

ACUPRESSURE/ACUPUNCTURE THERAPY

Acupressure and acupuncture are non-medicinal ways to help control pain. Acupressure uses pressure rather than needles to treat key areas of the body. Acupressure can be performed by the individual or a friend by applying pressure with the middle finger or thumb to acupressure points. A physical therapist, massage therapist, chiropractor or physician may have the training for acupressure treatment.

Acupuncture is a form of Chinese medicine in which inserting fine needles into the skin of the ear, the feet or other body parts relieves chronic pain, fatigue or other neurological symptoms. Pain relieving brain chemicals called endorphins and enkephalins are released during acupuncture. These chemicals block the pain circuits from sending their message to the brain so "you don't feel the pain." Acupuncture has few side effects if disposable, standard needles are used and are administered by a trained acupuncturist. Pain relief should be felt within 5-10 treatments. Physician acupuncturists and licensed acupuncturists are qualified to administer this treatment.

OTHER

Naturopathic, homeopathic, herbal and magnetic approaches to treatment have been helpful for some individuals.

WHAT CAN A PAIN CLINIC DO TO HELP?

In certain situations an inpatient or outpatient pain clinic may be an appropriate treatment approach. A team approach with the patient and their family as the center includes medical specialities of physical therapy, occupational therapy, vocational rehabilitation, psychology, nutrition, and physician. The goal is to enable the individual to return to daily activities of self care, family interaction, social interaction and to the vocational/work situation. The effective pain clinic works within the individual's limits, to develop coping skills, to develop and implement self care skills for pain and fatigue and to prescribe appropriate nonaddictive medications. Appropriate medications can enable the FMS individual to increase his/her endurance, strength, and daily activities initially in a controlled environment, then on an independent basis in society.

A typical daily routine in a pain clinic modified for the FMS individual might be:

8:00 a.m. hot shower and gentle stretching, breakfast
9:00 a.m. physiological quieting
9:30 a.m. stretching with breathing; overall body strengthening using theraband
10:15 a.m. rest cycle with biofeedback, snack
10:30 a.m. lifting, carrying, standing, sitting tolerance, vocational skill modification
11:30 a.m. rest cycle with quieting music
11:45 a.m. lunch with nutritional education

1:00 p.m. aerobic pool exercise or stationary bike or treadmill
stretches in hot tub

2:00 p.m. group therapy, behavior modification

3:15 p.m. rest period, snack
3:30 p.m. physical therapy modalities, massage
4:15 p.m. structured leisure activities
5:00 p.m. dinner

Initial evaluation and goal setting by the interdisciplinary team and weekly reassessment individualizes the treatment schedule. The questions are:

1. What can I do and have tolerable pain levels? What skills can help me with pain and fatigue?

2. What medications at what levels can help?

3. How can I approach work, home, family and leisure activities in a healthy way?

4. How can I learn to rest effectively at night and throughout the day?

5. How can I float through life's activities and stressors instead of being a bull in a china closet?

CHAPTER 8

WHAT CAN BIOFEEDBACK DO TO HELP?

Gail E. Nevin, P.T.
Janet A. Hulme, P.T.

Biofeedback measures and displays information occurring within the body, information about body temperature (circulation to muscles), muscle tension (electrical activity of muscles), heart rate, and emotional response. This is information that a person normally doesn't perceive, information that is at an unconscious level. Biofeedback enables an individual to be aware of these processes at a conscious level. Circulation, muscle activity and breathing patterns are commonly altered in FMS, so with accurate information/feedback about these areas, the individual with FMS can learn the feeling of a normal activity level. Frequently returning to that base line throughout the day is the basis for experiencing a more pain-free, fatigue-free daily life. The person with FMS gains back control over body functions that otherwise limit quality of life, daily social interactions and vocational capabilities. Biofeedback gives fast, accurate audio or visual information about body signals normally ignored or not consciously perceived.

In FMS, blood circulation to muscles of the back, arms, legs, hands and feet is often significantly decreased. Biofeedback can give accurate surface temperature information so FMS individuals can retrain blood vessels to dilate and increase blood flow to a body part.

Feedback about minute by minute, hour by hour breathing is not typically at a conscious level, whether an individual has FMS or not. The diaphragm, the major breathing muscle, is often significantly affected in FMS and accessory muscles of the neck and upper chest take over. Electromyography (EMG) biofeedback gives accurate measurable information about diaphragmatic and accessory muscle activity during breathing which then can enable the FMS individual to reeducate the diaphragm and accessory muscles and restore normal function.

In the FMS individual's muscles, the resting level in sitting, standing, or reclining is generally high. The brain center's perception of the muscle resting level is that it is normal, quiet and relaxed. EMG biofeedback gives accurate, immediate information to the conscious brain centers about muscle resting level activity via the auditory and visual cortex. The messages sent back to the muscles from those brain centers can then be appropriate for decreasing excessive activity at rest. Biofeedback supplements the unconscious centers that are receiving and perceiving inaccurate information with more accurate perception of muscle activity through the conscious centers.

During daily activities such as cleaning, cooking, typing, even socializing the muscles used for these activities "overdo" or are at a higher level of activity than muscles of a non-FMS individual while accomplishing the same task. Surface EMG biofeedback gives information to the conscious brain centers so muscle activity can be modified via messages sent from the brain to the muscle fibers. The individual with

FMS learns initially to check in using biofeedback equipment and then later replaces the biofeedback unit with using internal sensation, assessing muscles before, during, and after physical activities. That information is used to alter excessive activity, to learn "floating" techniques with the accurate information from external or internal biofeedback.

Biofeedback is also helpful in obtaining accurate information about and making changes in the response of the individual to stressors in daily life. The response of the FMS individual's heart, stomach, intestines, blood vessels, sweat glands etc. during daily stressors tends to be excessive. These organs overactivate.

Sleep disruption and fatigue are another major component of FMS. When there is a lack of effective sleep in FMS there is an inability of the body to repair and replace cell structures of all organ systems. Biofeedback is an important tool to assist the individual in consciously learning the patterns his/her body uses during rest and sleep, i.e., the muscle activity present, the breathing patterns used, the circulation changes present.

Biofeedback is often essential for FMS individuals to use so they can learn what normal equilibrium is, what a normal physiological base line for muscles and internal organ functions is. Returning to that base line frequently throughout the day is the basis for a return to relatively pain-free, fatigue-free, daily life. Returning to that base line throughout the day means daily activities are accomplished with muscular and organ efficiency and with a return to resting base line soon after a daily activity so energy can be conserved and utilized throughout the day instead of only for a short time. Efficiency and effectiveness of sleep functions enables the individual to restore energy and capability for the following day.

CHAPTER 9

WHAT CAN PSYCHOTHERAPY DO TO HELP?

Ellen S. Silverglat, M.S.W.
Janet A. Hulme, P.T.

Counseling and/or psychotherapy can be of help in several areas including transitional issues, career/life planning, issues of lost function, spiritual direction and psychological testing. Counseling occurs in individual, couple, family, or group settings. Different types of counseling include cognitive-behavioral, regression therapy, hypnosis, and spiritual counseling.

The person with FMS experiences numerous transitions accepting the condition and the changes it brings in self image, physical activity and time management. Living with a condition which is of indefinite duration is hard and until one can learn to think of time in more manageable quantities, it can be overwhelming. Talking with a person experienced in adjustment to chronic disease broadens the FMS individual's focus to include more than losses and negative change. Refocusing on positive aspects, what treatment can help and how to plan for both short and long term goals can diminish the feeling of hopelessness.

An illness that has no clear cut and predictable course really makes an individual feel out of control. In counseling, time is spent on rediscovering what you can do, how to make the "to do" list manageable, and what goals are realistic . . . all of which contribute to the feeling of regaining control and improved self esteem.

Counseling can help by addressing the global anxiety periodically experienced in FMS. The FMS individual may worry, "How can I make it through today? How will things be in the future?" Counseling teaches specific techniques to decrease anxiety that are very helpful in FMS.

Counseling assists in the treatment of depression that is common when there is significant long term pain. FMS individuals experience depression secondary to the chronic sleep disturbance, pain and fatigue. Some FMS individuals have a secondary diagnosis of clinical depression. In either case, the individual can be assisted by a psychotherapist and depression is treatable.

Psychological testing for memory problems and learning deficits can define the areas and extent of learning and processing problems and develop adaptations for school and work environments.

Counseling, especially cognitive-behavioral therapy, can help with accommodating changes in daily and weekly schedules. Cognitive-behavioral therapy teaches coping skills that help individuals control thoughts and actions that affect pain.

Regression therapy can assist the FMS individual in identifying early life events and family interactions that can be affecting how the person responds to daily life in the present.

Clinical hypnosis engages in a safe deep relaxation process, reaching a state of heightened awareness much like the edge of sleep, accessing the ability of the individual to reduce pain and fatigue.

Spiritual counseling involves pastoral assistance in the healing process.

A counselor, psychotherapist, psychiatrist or psychologist will assist in keeping things in perspective and help avoid seeing a catastrophe when a transient setback is what has happened.

Counseling is provided by certified or licensed mental health counselors, social workers, pastoral counselors, psychologists, and psychiatrists. In choosing a counselor it is important to interview the professional making sure they are educated about FMS, are compatible with the FMS individual, and interested in the same goals.

Group counseling can be very helpful and is often what occurs in support groups.

SUPPORT GROUPS

A support group can provide a sense of community for FMS individuals, a place to share the feelings, complaints, successes, treatments, and new research with others having the same chronic symptoms. A support group is also valuable for family members so they can gain information about the syndrome and begin to realize the encompassing symptoms as well as the variability and chronicity of FMS.

Newly diagnosed individuals can share feelings and questions with others who have experienced the fears and frustrations as well as the pain and fatigue. More experienced FMS individuals meet to share the latest management ideas, support each other in self care and provide emotional encouragement when there are exacerbations.

Support groups can organize calling circles or sponsors so anyone who needs it has a contact by phone when support is needed. Support groups often meet monthly for 1-2 hours utilizing part of the time for educational purposes and the rest for sharing between individuals.

Support groups, as they are active longer, can share information with the wider community through the print, radio, and TV media. They can also share with the health care community, government agencies and insurance companies through newsletters and workshops.

A new approach to support groups is through the computer internet. There is presently a fibromyalgia digest group on the NET. Physicians answer questions and individuals share useful management information.

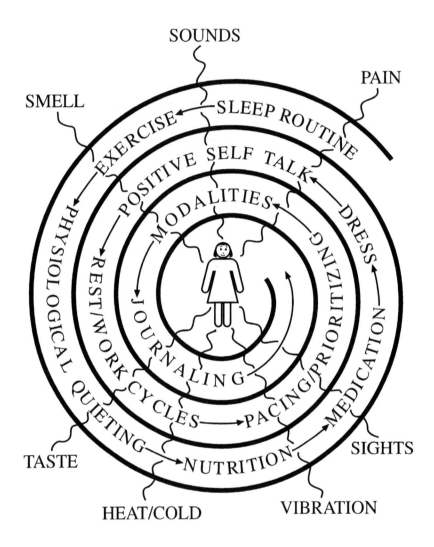

SOUNDS

PAIN

SMELL

SLEEP ROUTINE

EXERCISE

POSITIVE SELF TALK

MODALITIES

DRESS

PHYSIOISIOLOGICAL QUIETING

REST/WORK CYCLES

JOURNALING

PACING/PRIORITIZING

MEDICATION

TASTE

NUTRITION

SIGHTS

HEAT/COLD

VIBRATION

© J Hulme 1996

Figure 4: Daily Life Style Changes

PART III - WHAT CAN I DO TO STAY ACTIVE AND HEALTHY?

CHAPTER 10

WHAT CAN I DO TO TAKE CARE OF MYSELF?

Joyce Dougan, P.T.
Barbara Penner, P.T.
Gail E. Nevin, P.T.
Janet A. Hulme, P.T.

Self care centers around quieting/inhibiting exaggerated sensory input by making daily life style changes (Figure 4). Life style changes help normalize the FMS individual's hormonal and neurological communication systems. The individual can then be involved in work, play, family and social activities with ease and energy. The self care strategies are prioritized beginning with sleep protocols, exercise and physiological quieting. These are essential foundations for the FMS individual's health and well-being. It is recommended that an individual progress with the other self care skills gradually, adding a new one as the previous ones become more automatic and easy. It is not necessary to do everything at once.

SLEEP PROTOCOL

Since restful sleep is a top priority for FMS individuals, planning an individual routine for sleep is important. "I want to be able to get to sleep, sleep through the night without pain and frequent waking. I want to feel rested and limber when I awake."

To get to sleep:

1. Remove stimulants such as caffeine from your diet. This includes any coffee, tea, soda or chocolate that contains caffeine. Some headache and pain remedies contain caffeine and should be changed to another non-caffeine containing medication. Caffeine is a stimulant to the autonomic nervous system, increasing pain perception, stimulating the brain's arousal systems and facilitating wakefulness. It is also a bladder irritant so it can increase the times you need to go to the bathroom at night.

2. Hunger and/or hypoglycemia can increase insomnia symptoms so eating a light carbohydrate snack like a piece of whole wheat toast or a banana along with a small amount of a milk product just before bedtime can improve sleep. Milk products contain tryptophan, a natural chemical that has a calming and relaxing affect on the nervous system and is a precursor to serotonin. Milk products also contain calcium which helps with sleep and muscle relaxation. Carbohydrates help speed tryptophan to the brain.

3. A regular bedtime and wake up time is important for individuals with sleep disturbance. Eight to ten hours of sleep each night is important. Growth hormone in FMS individuals is produced in greatest amounts during the early morning hours, so the best sleep for FMS is sometimes termed "sleeping in" by others. Growth hormone is essential for growth and repair of all body cells. Shift changes at a job are not conducive to health with FMS individuals since the

body clock needs to practice the same routine over a long period of time and is hypersensitive to disruption.

4.   The hour before bedtime needs to be a time of winding down, a time for yourself and quiet enjoyment. It is not a time to be balancing the checkbook, paying the bills, or settling a family disagreement. Try soft music, a hot bath, a good book, or writing in a journal. This is the time to use physiological quieting in preparation for sleep.

To stay asleep:

1.   Use a supportive mattress that has its own soft pad or place an egg crate mattress under the sheet and mattress pad. Try different pillows until you find the best one for your head and neck, one that is most comfortable through the night and enables you to wake up with the minimum of stiffness and soreness in your neck and shoulders. Use a pillow between your knees and hug one when you sleep on your side. When sleeping on your back, place pillows under your knees as well as supporting your head and neck. You may even want pillows to support each shoulder and arm. Sleeping on your stomach is not recommended because of the extreme position it puts your neck and low back.

2.   Wear warm night wear with long sleeves and long pants. Some people even wear socks, gloves and nightcaps to help maintain body temperature while sleeping.

3.   Warm the bed before you get in using a heating pad or electric mattress pad. Turn it off before you go to sleep.

4.   Eliminate environmental factors that can arouse a light sleeper. Dark out shades and a sleep mask keep out light. A sound conditioner which produces white noise or ear plugs block out the background noise of car engines, horns, and people talking. Essential oils such as birch, and lemon can facilitate restfulness and block out other stimulating smells. Stabilize the room heat so the temperature is the same all

night and use blankets which are adequate for the duration of sleep.

5. Exercise moderately 20-30 minutes some time during the day at least three hours before bedtime. Exercising in the evening stimulates the nervous system and may increase alertness and wakefulness.

6. If you wake up during the night move to a comfortable position, then relax muscles, head to toe, into the bed and begin diaphragmatic breathing, hand warming, and positive self statements. Know that your body and mind are in a restful state even if you do not perceive that you are asleep.

7. If you can't get back to sleep after a half an hour to an hour get up, read a book, write in a journal, or do some gentle exercise, and then try to sleep again later.

8. Use prescribed medication consistently. Consult a physician about changes in sleep patterns.

The goal: SLEEP THROUGH THE NIGHT, WAKE RESTED AND LIMBER!

EXERCISE

Exercise in moderation is essential to optimum function for FMS individuals. Exercise guidelines are described in Chapter 11.

PHYSIOLOGICAL QUIETING

Each individual responds to events in daily life through biochemical changes within the body and brain. The alarm in the morning is perceived by the ear, transferred to the brain center for hearing by biochemical events within the nerve, then interpreted by the brain centers which send messages to the rest of the body through additional chemicals saying, "open your eyes, jump out of bed, get dressed." Chemicals are different depending on how the event is perceived by the brain. If the event is perceived as an emergency, fight or flight event, chemicals such as adrenaline and testosterone are released in increased amounts; if the event is perceived as a normal, easy life event the brain and body chemicals are different and give activating but calmer directions to all organs and tissues.

FMS individuals' brain centers and nervous systems tend to respond to life events with fight or flight chemicals rather than quieting chemicals. The autonomic or automatic nervous system that controls heart rate, breathing, stomach and intestine activity, bladder function, and circulation tends to send out more fight or flight chemicals than quieting chemicals. We say it has a high idle at rest, always ready to jump. The on/off switch for full activation is hypersensitive. This means even normal daily events may activate biochemicals that are meant only for use during short periods of high stress. This constant activation of stress chemicals is destructive to the body over the long term. Circulation to muscles is decreased so muscles ache from lack of oxygen and accumulation of waste products. Breathing rate increases and breathing is shallow and irregular so the FMS individual complains of shortness of breath and low endurance during aerobic activity. Heart rate increases and is often irregular, chest pain and pressure are experienced. Stomach and intestinal activity increases, excessive abnormal smooth muscle contractions can cause stomach and abdominal pain, diarrhea, and indigestion. Hyperalertness occurs and light irregular sleep patterns prevent repair and replacement of all body cells.

It is important to use management techniques that quiet the high idle or high resting level of the nervous system. It is important to use management techniques that assist the autonomic nervous system in responding to daily events with "calm" chemical activation of organ systems instead of "fight or flight" emergency activation.

These techniques are termed PHYSIOLOGICAL QUIETING. They are management techniques targeted to the autonomic nervous system. The three major techniques are:

1. BREATHING
2. HAND WARMING
3. BODY/MIND QUIETING

BREATHING

Approximately ten to fifteen percent of FMS individuals have a sense of dyspnea (air hunger) even in a resting state. During exercise an FMS individual's breathing pattern is irregular when normal individuals would have extremely regular breathing. The diaphragm, the major breathing muscle, becomes dysfunctional much as other muscles do in FMS. Accessory breathing muscles in the neck and chest take over for the diaphragm. Since breathing affects tissue oxygen levels, body metabolism, heart rate and the body's acid base balance, when breathing is erratic and the muscle action producing breathing patterns is changed, these physiological processes are severely altered. Heart rate is increased, nerve/ muscle resting level is elevated, and blood pressure changes. Symptoms described by FMS individuals that can be directly attributed to hyperventilation, the most drastic form of erratic breathing, include: dyspnea, palpitations, chest pain, choking or smothering sensation, dizziness, vertigo, paresthesia, hot and cold flashes, faintness, trembling, and fear or anxiety feelings. With this in mind, returning to diaphragmatic breathing becomes an important aspect of FMS management.

The diaphragm is a large sheetlike muscle that rests in a dome shape upward into the chest to the nipple area from the bottom of the rib cage and the spine. As you inhale the dome flattens and pulls down to the bottom of the rib cage. During exhale the diaphragm moves back to the dome shape. When breathing correctly, the shoulder and chest areas remain quiet, the jaw is relaxed, and the teeth are separated. Inhale, let your abdomen rise, exhale, let it fall. There is equal time for inhale and exhale, inhaling through the nose, exhaling through the mouth or nose. Exhale is passive and quiet.

Diaphragmatic breathing eases and reverses the biochemical effects of hyperventilation and makes it easier for air to flow into the lungs. Practice the diaphragmatic breathing initially in a reclined position, then in sitting and standing. Practice hourly during the day, 7-8 breaths.

HAND WARMING

Circulation to muscles, nerves, internal organs, and the brain is often significantly decreased in FMS individuals. FMS individuals describe being core cold, not being able to warm up. Their hands and feet are cold, their buttocks feel cold, even their internal organs feel cold. Often a cold feeling is a cardinal sign of worsening FMS symptoms of muscle aching and fatigue within the next 6-8 hours.

Decreased circulation means blood vessel constriction. Blood vessel walls have three layers, one of which is muscular. The muscular layer is controlled by the sympathetic (fight or flight) nervous system. An active sympathetic system causes constriction of the blood vessel wall, a quieting sympathetic system causes dilation or relaxation of the blood vessel wall, so the blood vessels allow more blood flow. When more blood flows through the vessels there is increased heat from the increased blood volume which results in hands, feet and other body parts warming.

Hand warming is a technique to increase blood volume to body parts. Mental imaging and frequently repeated thoughts transfer to nerve activity that quiets the sympathetic (fight or flight) nervous system activity resulting in dilation of blood vessels. To accomplish this:

1. "Visualize the warmest place your hands can be, holding a warm cup of hot chocolate, holding your hands over a camp fire or radiator, or slipping your hands and feet in the hot sand of a beach on a summer day."

2. "Think of the warmest color and surround your hands and wrists with that color. Let that color flow into your hands, deep into the palms, fingers, wrists while they get warmer and warmer."

3. "Focus your attention to your hands and say to yourself, "My hands are warmer and warmer, warmth is flowing into my hands, warmer and warmer. "

To accomplish a resetting of the autonomic nervous system, to slow the high idle, it is necessary to practice the techniques that quiet the sympathetic system frequently for short periods. The instructions are: "Practice hourly for 30-60 seconds, wherever you are. No one will know you are doing it." Put colored dots up around your work and home or buy a watch that buzzes every hour to remind you. Then hourly do:

- 7-8 slow, low diaphragmatic breaths
- Release jaw, quiet shoulders, quiet chest
- 7-8 repetitions of hand warming

BODY / MIND QUIETING

Body/mind quieting serves many important functions in helping FMS individuals. Excessive muscle resting levels and internal organ activity can be decreased through physiological quieting of the body/mind. Abnormal sleep patterns are improved with physiological quieting of the body/mind. Physiological quieting of the body/mind assists the immune system in optimal functioning.

To accomplish body/mind quieting:

Find a quiet, warm room with a chair or bed that gives complete support from your head to your feet. Use pillows for support of your neck, low back, arms, and knees.

1. Focus on your breathing, feel the pattern of breathing, let your abdomen rise with inhale, fall with exhale.

2. Feel the warmth or coolness of your hands and feet, left side and right. Let your hands and feet feel warm, feel warmer and warmer.

3. Feel the support of the bed or chair and release into that support, let your feet, legs, hips, back, shoulders, arms, neck and head sink deeper and deeper into that support.

4. Focus on your face and neck. Notice where there is any tension or tightness, where there is quiet, calmness in each part of your face and neck muscles – your forehead, eyes, cheeks, tongue, throat, neck. Then say to yourself 3-4 times slowly, "My face and neck muscles are quiet and calm, my face and neck muscles are calmer and calmer."

5. Proceed from head to toe in the same manner, focusing on head and neck, back (upper, middle and lower), shoulders and arms, hips and legs, chest and abdomen.

6. Focus again on diaphragmatic breathing, and hand warming.

One to two 20 minute body/mind quieting sessions a day are recommended. Try doing it 20 minutes before you get out of bed in the morning and 20 minutes before going to sleep at night. The Physiological Quieting audiotape is available through Phoenix Publishing.

Integrating physiological quieting throughout the day is an essential aspect of self care in FMS management.

NUTRITION

Certain foods, vitamins, or allergies to foods or chemicals do not cause fibromyalgia. Individuals may find specific foods that seem to exacerbate symptoms and others that seem to help. In general, any food or drink that is an irritant to the nervous system may exacerbate symptoms. For example, the caffeine in coffee, tea, soda and chocolate is a nervous system irritant and aggravates symptoms of muscle pain, sleep disturbance, and bladder irritability. On the other hand, food or drink that has a quieting affect may help decrease symptoms. For example, the high fiber in complex carbohydrates may quiet irritable bowel symptoms.

FMS individuals may have hypoglycemic tendencies. This means their blood sugar levels vary with extremes on the low end that give them a feeling of weakness, irritability, and disorientation. Staying away from sugars and eating small meals 5-6 times a day instead of three bigger meals can help minimize these symptoms. Eating long acting complex carbohydrates such as green beans, apples, cereal or cookies containing oatmeal and whole wheat breads with adequate protein can also help in maintaining blood glucose levels.

Adequate consumption of water and noncaffeinated fluids is important for a FMS individual's health. The increased accumulation of waste products in muscle and connective tissues increases pain and pressure feelings. Adequate fluid consumption, 6-8 glasses per day, helps the circulatory system and kidneys process waste products.

When eating meals or snacks it is important to watch portion sizes, especially of protein and fat. Thin slices of cheese and "deck of cards" size meat portions are adequate for nutritional needs. Hunger can be satisfied with carbohydrates, fruits and vegetables instead of increased fat.

Some FMS individuals try to eat fatigue and achiness away. A common thought is, "If I just eat something I'll have more energy or not hurt as much." In other instances, when feelings of despair or depression are prevalent, the idea that food is a comforter leads to excessive calories being consumed. It is true that food can be quieting and comforting. Carbohydrates, for instance, tend to soothe the nervous system and gut. Yet it is important to recognize the symptoms and treat the pain, fatigue or depression, not try to cover them up or numb the senses with food.

It is vital to eat and drink adequately while exercising. Before starting an exercise program eat a light carbohydrate meal and drink 6-8 oz. of fluid. During workouts drink fluids every 10-15 minutes. It is important to consume a high carbohydrate meal with protein within 15-20 minutes after exercise to replenish energy stores.

There are indications of decreased blood or muscle cell levels of magnesium in FMS individuals. Five hundred milligrams of magnesium daily is recommended by some experts.

Other vitamins and minerals that are important in a daily dietary plan for FMS include:

Vitamin C – 500 to 3000 mg/day

Vitamin Bs – 25-50 mg/day

Calcium – 800 - 1000 mg/day for females premenopause,
    1200-1500 mg/day menopause or post menopause
    (300 mg = 8 oz. milk or 1 slice cheese)

Vitamin E – 200-400 IU/day

Vitamin D – 20 minutes of sunlight/day

Malic Acid – 1200-1400 mg/day

SIX TO EIGHT GLASSES OF WATER DAILY!
(decaffeinated fluids)

Vitamin C is present in citrus fruits and functions as an antioxidant, it may have antibiotic-like qualities at higher doses, and assists the intestines in normal functioning. Vitamin B complex, present in green leafy vegetables, is essential for nerve transmission and healthy functioning of the nerves and liver. It affects sleep, mental capacity, heart and lung functions. Vitamin E, present in brown rice, kale, apricots, sunflower and pumpkin seeds, can improve circulation and cellular function. Magnesium, present in green leafy vegetables, legumes and nuts, is essential for muscle and heart functioning. It inhibits action of excitatory amino acids that lead to increased pain and discomfort. Magnesium levels are inversely related to pain/tenderness levels, the higher the magnesium levels in muscle cells, the lower the pain complaints. Calcium, present in milk products, is essential for muscle function as well as bone strength. Calcium-magnesium combination is an effective muscle relaxant. Malic acid is a food acid present in apples and other fruits. It is important for cell function and energy production in cells. It can be obtained as magnesium malate.

OPTIMIZE MEDICATIONS

Medications are often recommended as part of the total management approach for FMS. Medications rarely eliminate all symptoms but often help with the sleep disorder and to decrease pain. To find the optimum medication combination, it may take the physician several trials of different drugs and amounts. Medication can be used over months and even years so a medication may lose its effectiveness after a period of time and need to be changed for another. Know what characteristics each medication has, its side effects, and how and when it should be taken. If there is more than one physician prescribing medication be sure each knows all the medications being taken so combinations don't cause serious side effects. There are prescription guides available in bookstores or at the pharmacy to help you stay informed.

One last word about medication. Since FMS is a chronic condition, medications that help are frequently needed over an extended period of time and on a daily basis. There is a tendency for FMS individuals to take medication until they feel better and then quit taking it or take it infrequently. "I don't want to be dependent on drugs to feel good. I'm not someone who uses drugs," are commonly heard comments. The mental set that is needed when thinking about FMS and medications is that the individual has a lack of certain chemicals that then increase the fatigue and pain. The medications help replace those missing chemicals so the body can function optimally. They are often needed over the long term to help the FMS individual experience the fewest symptoms.

DRESS

The clothing a person wears makes a statement about personal style, helps with temperature regulation and offers protection. The FMS individual benefits from layered clothing so pieces can be added or subtracted as temperature changes. Air conditioning often increases FMS symptoms so light turtle necks and long sleeve shirts or sweaters are needed for protection in that environment. During winter weather silk or other light weight but warm underwear is often needed under all types of clothing. Glove and boot warmers are helpful if the person is going to be out in the cold weather. Tight, binding clothing is not tolerated when FMS symptoms include skin hypersensitivity or tender point pain in an area. Soft fabrics, elasticized waists, and sports bras will be more comfortable than tight, form fitting items. Supportive, well fitting shoes rather than slip on, high heel shoes are essential for daily life and the work environment. Walking or running shoes that have maximum cushioning are usually the best. Warm socks or slippers instead of bare feet are best at home.

SELF TALK – POSITIVE SELF STATEMENTS

The mind is always saying something positive, negative,

or neutral as an individual goes through the day. Even while sleeping at night there are thoughts and dreams. Self talk, or positive self statements, can be helpful or hurtful in relation to FMS symptoms and an individual's accomplishments. To develop an awareness of what self talk is like, for one or two days pause four or five times during the day and jot down what thoughts are present at that time in relation to what the FMS individual is doing and how he/she is feeling. Are there primarily positive or negative thoughts? Are there repetitive thoughts? Now take the positive thoughts and repeat them throughout the day such as every time breathing practice is scheduled or every time the individual talks on the phone. Pair the positive self statement with some event that occurs frequently in the day. If there is negative self talk, substitute positive statements for the negative thoughts.

Examples of positive self statements are:
1 . I am healing, I am healing more each moment of each day.
2. I am trying, I am doing the best I can.
3 . I deserve to be healthy and happy, I am healthy and happy.
4. I feel quiet and calm, I am quiet and calm.
5. I love you, I will take care of you.

For some individuals positive self statements seem like lies or half truths. If that occurs, put "I am trying" or "I am beginning to" in front of the statement. Remember every thought is a biochemical event in the brain and body which then has an effect on all other body and mind functions.

REST IS A TREATMENT ESSENTIAL IN FMS

Rest is a vital part of anyone's daily schedule, usually accomplished at an unconscious level. Relaxing into a chair for a few minutes between jobs, reading the newspaper or watching television and dozing off for a short period, sitting under a tree and gazing at the clouds during lunch time, and sitting at your desk stretching towards the ceiling while releasing two or three big sighs are all forms of rest the body and mind need and ask for throughout the day. Rest is necessary for energy conservation and a return to neutrality or to slow idle before going on to a new task.

Both mind and body rest are important to accomplish during the slow idle periods throughout the day. Mind rest techniques can include meditation, positive self talk, and breathing awareness to name a few. Body rest includes skeletal muscle release and internal organ systems' quieting using physiological quieting techniques such as breathing and hand warming. The need for supportive, comfortable chairs, couches and beds that enable the individual's muscles to let go into a relaxed state with minimal pain are important for body rest as well.

Mind and body rest needs to occur frequently throughout the day for short periods. Sometimes it will only be a minute or so of breathing and quiet muscle release, other times 5 minutes of focused meditation, and at least 20-30 minutes of extended mind and body rest using physiological quieting techniques once a day. When setting up a schedule for the day, REST PERIODS are as important as work periods. These rest periods help ensure that the FMS tendency for elevated resting levels of muscle activity, autonomic nervous system activity and mental activity are frequently returned to more normal levels, to a slow idle. Then there can be conservation of energy to be used throughout the day instead of only for short bursts followed by exhaustion. These rest periods can be essential in maintaining a decreased pain and fatigue level throughout the day instead of the pattern of a small window of relief in the morning and escalating pain and fatigue levels the remainder of the day.

PACING – ENERGY MANAGEMENT

Pacing is the breaking up of the day into multiple work, rest, and play sections. To pace the day it is important to first make a list of the work related tasks for the day and prioritize the top three while putting off till tomorrow the others. Pacing is breaking each of those jobs or tasks into two or three parts with planned rest periods in between.

Pacing is not finishing one job before you start a part of another one. Instead it means performing the first part of job one, then resting, then going to the first part of job two, then resting, then completing the first part of job three, then resting, then going back to the second part of job one, etc. With this kind of pacing, different muscles and different body postures are used for each new job so that fatigue is not such a problem because parts of jobs are done with frequent changes in muscle action and postural alignment. The idea is that frequent short rest periods with conscious return to neutral mind and body activity enables the FMS individual to accomplish more tasks with less fatigue and pain.

DAILY JOB LIST   DAILY PRIORITY JOBS

1. Sweep floors   1. Sweep floors
2.   a. part one: Sweep ½ kitchen floor
3.   b. part two: Sweep ½ kitchen floor
4.   c. part three: Sweep laundry room
5.   2.
6.   a. part one:
7.   b. part two:
                        c. part three:
                     3.
                        a. part one:
                        b. part two:
                        c. part three:

REST ACTIVITIES
1. Listening to music while reclining.
2. Reading in supported sitting.
3. Physiologic quieting.
4. Diaphragmatic breathing and hand warming.

Initially the rest cycles may be longer than work cycles, but gradually the two will become equal and eventually the work cycle can exceed the rest cycle and still maintain the goals of decreased pain and fatigue. For example:

Rest Cycle	Work Cycle
10 minutes	3-5 minutes
	increase 1-2 minutes/week
10 minutes	10 minutes
10 minutes	15 minutes

Pacing means placing play and laughter into the work, rest routine throughout the day, not just when all work has been accomplished. PLAY AND LAUGHTER ARE REQUIRED TREATMENTS MULTIPLE TIMES DURING EACH DAY. With that being the case, short periods of play will be scheduled into mid morning, mid afternoon, and evening. On some occasions, segments can be as simple and short as reading the funnies in the paper every morning and making sure to practice belly laughing. There needs to be a daily 20-30 minute play period with friends over tea, or spending 20 minutes in a hot bath or hot tub, going to the movie, or watching a favorite TV program.

Some individuals, when asked what they do for fun, respond "work." It is necessary to begin making a master list of play and fun activities that are not work related so you can vary the play activities on a daily and weekly basis and continue to be on the lookout for a new play or fun activity to add to the list. Try to find a new one every week or two. Watch other people and catch them having fun, see what they are doing. It means that play and laughter have equal weight with work and rest in a daily schedule.

Pacing of work, rest and play can be easily monitored by using a daily journal. As part of a nightly routine fill in the day's activities and summarize where pacing went well.

DAILY JOURNAL OF PLAY, REST, WORK

Time	Play	Rest	Work
			(ea. task = 3 parts)
			(3-4 tasks/day)
A.M. 7:00-8:00			
8:00-9:00			
9:00-10:00			

PLAY ACTIVITY LIST
1. Tea with friends
2. Favorite video
3. Reading the funnies
4. Soaking in the bath or hot tub
5.

PRIORITIZING
Prioritizing is making decisions – decisions that some work is more important to do today, that some work is more important to do next week and some work you should never do but rather give to someone else or let it go undone. Prioritizing is listing all the work titles you have and the roles you carry out under each of those, then making

decisions as to which are important to be done on a daily, weekly, monthly or never ever basis. It needs to be emphasized that prioritizing is done in the context of the pacing schedule you have already planned. PRIORITIZING IS MORE IMPORTANT THAN GETTING ALL YOUR JOB ROLES ACCOMPLISHED. FIGURE OUT HOW THE JOB ROLES CAN FIT INTO YOUR OPTIMUM PACING SCHEDULE.

WORK TITLES I FULFILL	**ROLES**
Examples:	
1. Parent to children	1. Transporter
2. Parent to elderly parents (list specifics)	2. House cleaner
3. Spouse	3. Listener/emotional support
4. Banker, teacher, teller etc.	4. Money transfer, reaching, grasp
5. Volunteer	
6. Friend	

PAIN RELIEVING MODALITIES

Pain relief is the number one priority for most individuals with fibromyalgia. Effective techniques may be different for each person. Examples of pain relieving modalities include:

HEAT

The benefits from 20-30 minutes of heat include increased circulation and decreased muscle tightness. Moist heat pads are usually preferred over dry heating pads. The moist heating pad purchased at the drug store will often have little sponges that are moistened. Medical supply stores have heating pads that draw moisture from the air. They are a little more costly but are larger and conform better to the body contours. A

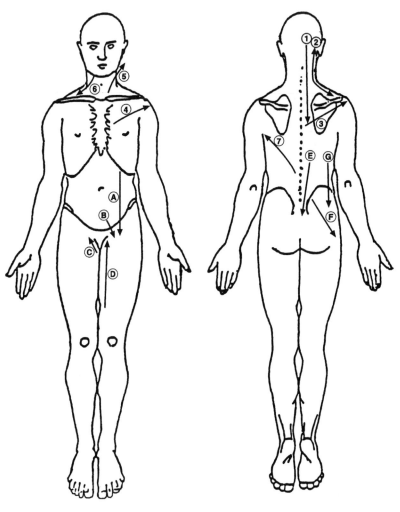

Figure 5: Fluoromethane Spray Techniques

© J Hulme 1996

damp towel or commercial hot pack heated in the microwave or in hot water for a few minutes is another good way to get moist heat. Hot water in the form of a hot tub, hot shower, or whirlpool bath is always a good choice. Hot tubs need to be under 102°F to allow an individual to stay in the water comfortably and safely for 20-30 minutes.

COLD

Some individuals benefit from ice so it is worth a try even if it sounds uncomfortable. One form of treatment is an ice massage to a painful area. Freeze water in an 8 oz. paper cup, then tear away the top edge of paper so the ice can be moved around the palm size painful area for about five minutes. Initially it feels very cold but within five minutes the area will be numb. Use a towel to catch the drips. Some individuals find it more tolerable to use ice while in a hot tub or shower or while they have heat on another part of the body. If cold hands are a problem, use gloves and a styrofoam cup.

An ice pack is another form of cold application. Commercial ice packs and ice probes are available through medical supply stores. Ice packs can be homemade using a wet or dry towel wrapped around a package of frozen peas or corn or crushed ice. A frozen wet towel provides more intense cold. A ten minute application of an ice pack is usually adequate.

FLUOROMETHANE SPRAY – HEAT

This technique is designed to obtain effective pain relief and increased motion in affected body areas. Fluoromethane spray is a cold, fine spray of fluoromethane gas under pressure. It is prescribed by a physician for clinic and/or home use. For use with FMS, body segments are treated instead of one or two specific muscles and the body position during the treatment is more midline than stretched as it is when myofascial muscle shortening is being treated. The term "midline spray and heat" is used rather than the more common term "spray and stretch." Initially a physician or therapist can use the technique as part of the office visit to evaluate effectiveness and improve pain and limited range of motion. If the technique is effective, the health care professional can demonstrate the techniques to a support person so the home program can be done 1-2 times daily during painful flare-ups (Figure 5). When pain is primarily in the upper body, (neck, shoulders, arms, shoulder blades, chest) the spray techniques 1-7 are completed bilaterally even though the pain and limited range of motion are present on only one side. When pain is primarily in the lower body, (low back, hips, buttocks, legs, abdomen) the spray techniques A-G are completed bilaterally.

ALTERNATE HEAT – ICE – HEAT

Some individuals get the most benefit from using a combination of heat and ice. Use heat (heating pad, hot tub) for 7-10 minutes, then cold (ice pack, ice probe) for 3-5 minutes, and then heat for 7-10 minutes.

HEAT – STRETCH AND ICE – HEAT

This technique is designed to obtain an effective stretch of a tight muscle group without setting off muscle spasms. Heat the muscle group for about three minutes, then put that area on a gentle stretch and hold the stretch while rubbing an ice cup or ice edge in lines about 1/2 inch apart parallel to the muscle fibers under the skin. Keep the stretch gentle and steady for 30-60 seconds then heat the area again for approximately three minutes.

MASSAGE

Self massage or having a family member massage areas can be effective using essential oils and light to moderate stroking over muscle areas that are painful or tight. The touch helps quiet and relax the muscles and the essential oils help increase circulation, decrease pain and tightness. It is important to avoid trying to "dig out" the pain with deep, intense massage techniques which will often increase the symptoms. The pain does not have to get worse before it can get better. Essential oils are always used in a carrier oil such as olive or almond oil. Tender point pressure, direct pressure using the thumb or a finger for 7-8 seconds is one beneficial technique. Direct pressure over acupressure sites for 7-8 seconds can be effective for pain relief and easy to do several times a day (Figure 6).

Using two tennis balls in a sock and putting the balls between the individual and the floor to massage a particular spot for 1-3 minutes decreases pain. Two racket balls in a sock fit the base of the neck better than tennis balls. There are various canes and knobs on the market to help you reach difficult spots. Hiring a professional massage therapist for a weekly massage is also beneficial. Interview them first, make sure they understand the needs of fibromyalgia.

OILS AND LOTIONS

A number of lotions, creams and oils can be used in combination with medication to ease muscle pain and tightness. Especially for those individuals who are drug sensitive, oils and lotions don't cause stomach or gastrointestinal irritation or the side effects of some medications yet they can give relief from pain and muscle tightness.

Essential oil mixtures in a base oil such as almond oil can be easily applied to painful areas by the individual or

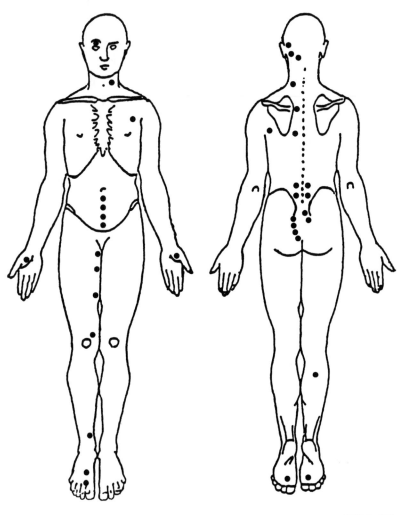

© J Hulme 1996

Figure 6: Acupressure Sites

76

family member. Specific oils decrease pain, detoxify waste products and improve circulation. Commonly used essential oils include lavender, lemon, rosemary, juniper, and bergamot.

Lotions containing capsaicin are known to decrease substance P. Capsaicin is derived from red peppers and produces a hot, burning sensation when rubbed into the skin. Repeated application to a specific area over a week can result in decreased pain. Other lotions produce a cooling effect on the skin for relief of pain and discomfort.

JOURNALING

The habit of regularly writing in a blank book or on pages in a notebook can be helpful in tracking the ups and downs of fibromyalgia, in seeing small steps of progress that lead to improved health, and in relieving the "free floating" anxiety FMS individuals describe.

Journaling is "stream of conscious" writing. There is no right or wrong way to do it. Just open the blank book or take some note paper and write whatever flows from the mind and hand. No one needs to read it or judge it. Let the mind empty all its thoughts, worries, and concerns on the paper. When the censor part of the mind tries to stop the thought flow to the paper, remember this writing is not for judging, it is for releasing feeling and thoughts.

In FMS at times the brain activity for thoughts, worries, and ideas becomes excessive, getting in the way of everyday life just as the muscles become overactive causing pain and fatigue. The overactive brain leads to feelings of anxiety, confusion, indecision, and mental paralysis. Releasing any and all thoughts to paper assists in quieting brain activity.

Journaling can be done day or night. Keep notebooks at a bed stand and in a purse. Some FMS individuals are not able to write so a computer or audio or video tape recorder is a better mode of communication.

It is common for FMS individuals to resist letting thoughts and feelings out onto paper. "I don't have time. This is stupid. I know what I think so why do I have to write it down?" are comments made. Mark had FMS and experienced unexplained anxiety. He reluctantly agreed to do journal entries for three weeks. He described hating the first week and having to force himself to write. During the second week he noticed his concerns and anxiety didn't take up as much of his day as they used to. He got out an old oil paint set and started painting again. He bought a new CD to listen to. At the end of the third week he laughingly said he no longer waited to be overcome by anxiety before writing pages. He now was journaling as a part of his morning routine before eating breakfast.

CRISIS MANAGEMENT PROGRAM

It can be helpful to keep a daily journal to pick up patterns and relationships between symptoms and daily activities and stressors. In the journal the FMS individual keeps track of pain, stiffness and fatigue levels during morning, noon, afternoon and evening, medication taken, menstrual cycle pattern, exercise level, and jobs done.

The goal for FMS individuals is to modify activities or stressors that increase symptoms so there is an equilibrium achieved for extended periods of time. The equilibrium is often not a completely pain-free state, nor totally fatigue-free, but interventions throughout the day keep the equilibrium. A self care routine with regular mini reassessments of mind-body function are essential to attain that steady state of equilibrium.

Flare-ups or exacerbations are going to occur in FMS even with the best management program. A prearranged crisis management plan that is posted in a convenient place will help the FMS individual deal with the flare-ups. The crisis management plan is comprised of items that have worked in the past in order of priority, a list of support people to contact, and positive self statements that direct the mind and body towards health and healing.

EXAMPLE OF CRISIS MANAGEMENT PLAN
Alter the day's plans to fit your needs!
1. Use modalities such as hot shower or hot tub for 20 minutes.
2. Take 20 minutes 2-3 times today for physiological quieting.
3. Use pain relieving oil or lotion on affected muscles.
4. Do breathing and hand warming every half hour to hour.
5. Take a relaxing walk with a friend.
6. Take medication as directed for crisis times.
7. Increase rest cycle length in the daily plan.
8. Emphasize positive self statements.
9. Evaluate life stressors, i.e., environmental, emotional.
10. Consult with therapist or physician if not improved in 48 hours.

POSTURE
Standing and sitting posture is the base from which movement occurs. In FMS during standing it is common to see forward head, elevated, rounded shoulders, hyper-extended knees and weight acceptance on one leg more than another. The shoulder and neck muscles are over active and seem to hold the body up. The head and shoulders often lead during walking.

It is important to understand that standing posture should be maintained primarily by the bony skeleton and ligaments, not muscle action. There is minimal activity of the ankle muscles to maintain balance but the shoulder muscles, the abdominal and buttocks muscles should be relaxed. To stand in the most effective pain-free posture:

1. Take weight equally on both feet.
2. Unlock both knees.
3. Center the pelvis over knees and feet.
4. Lift the chest up and out, thinking of a string gently pulling upward.
5. Release shoulders, thinking of the shoulder and neck muscles as a velvet cloak resting on a hangar (the skeleton).
6. Release jaw, teeth apart, tongue released from the roof of the mouth.
7. Glide the head back with the chin dropped slightly.
8. Lengthen the spine by thinking of a string pulling from the back of the top of the head towards the clouds. Let the chin drop slightly.
9. Slow, low diaphragmatic breathe in the low abdomen.

Once the standing posture is comfortable, progress to:

1. Weight shift in small amplitudes side to side.
2. Perform slow, small knee bends.
3. Weight shift front to back with one foot in front of the other.

During these exercises, lead with the hips, keeping the shoulders and neck released and relaxed. Maintain slow, low diaphragmatic breathing.

To sit in the most effective, pain-free posture:

1. Take weight equally on both feet.
2. Take weight equally on both hips.
3. Center pelvis over hips.
4. Lift chest up and out thinking of a string pulling upwards.
5. Release shoulders, thinking of the shoulder and neck muscles as a velvet cloak resting on a hangar (the skeleton).

6. Release jaw, teeth apart, tongue released from the roof of the mouth.

7. Glide the head back with the chin dropped slightly.

8. Lengthen the spine by thinking of a string pulling from the back of the top of the head up towards the clouds. Let the chin drop slightly.

9. Slow, low diaphragmatic breathe in low abdomen.

Once the sitting posture is comfortable, progress to the following exercises:

1. Weight shift from side to side, one hip to the other. Increase the distance between ribs and hip on the side taking the weight.

2. Weight shift front to back, rock the pelvis front to back over the thighs.

During these exercises, lead with the hips, keeping the shoulders and neck released and relaxed. Maintain slow, diaphragmatic breathing.

CHAPTER 11

WHAT CAN I DO
TO STAY PHYSICALLY FIT?

Joyce Dougan, P.T.
Barbara Penner, P.T.
Janet A. Hulme, P. T.

Physical fitness develops through regular exercise, 20 to 30 minutes daily as a maintenance dose. It becomes part of a routine like brushing your teeth or combing your hair. It may seem like an effort at first but eventually the individual with FMS does not want to miss it.

Start an exercise program with just a few activities and a few repetitions (three to five), then progress as tolerated. Be the tortoise and not the hare. It is better to successfully get to the finish line than start fast and burn out. Try to do a few activities several times a day rather than doing a lot at one time once a day. The more frequent exercise/stretches help keep the FMS individual from getting so sore and stiff throughout the day. It is also a good way to breakup sustained activities such as typing, sitting in class, driving, or standing.

Start out your morning with "stretch and yawn" while still in bed. This is doing what feels good, not a specific set of stretches. This is what small children do when they awaken

. . . be a kid again! Doing neck and upper back stretches works especially well in a hot shower. Doing shoulder shrugs and rolls, performing head rolls side to side, stretching arms forward and back, are simple activities that can be done seated or standing as a work break. They can be completed in less than a minute so work flow is not interrupted. In fact, the mini exercise routine will likely increase the individual's concentration and productivity.

A few stretches or exercises at lunch and coffee breaks help relax the muscles that have been used during work and increase blood flow to the area while decreasing tension. Another good time for the FMS individuals to take a few minutes for themselves is after work and before tackling the evening activities. When not working outside the home, it is important to develop a daily routine. In addition to bed and shower stretches, doing some stretches and exercises after breakfast, mid morning, after lunch and before dinner helps with pain and stiffness. Another approach is to set a timer and do exercises every two hours for 3-5 minutes.

STRETCHING
The goal of stretching is to increase the ease of pain-free movement. For the individual with FMS the technique for stretching a tight muscle is different than a "feel good" full motion stretch. The fibromyalga stretch is called midline stretching. Stretching needs to be done when the body is warm and relaxed. This can be accomplished in a hot shower, after a warm bath, after 5-10 minutes of heat application, or following active exercise. Muscles need to be stretched slowly just until the beginning of discomfort is noted. Breathe into the stretch for 15-30 seconds. Think slow, small, soft, smooth, sensitive stretch. The breath is low, diaphragmatic breathing. Stretching to "pull out" the tightness doesn't work. It can set off more muscle tightening. Return to neutral slowly

and smoothly to avoid rebound tightening. One to three repetitions is enough. The typical stretch to the end of range with overpressure sets off the already overactive stretch reflex and feeds into the high resting tone (gamma bias) present in FMS muscles.

STRENGTHENING

If the word strengthening brings to mind visions of Arnold Swartzenegger, don't be overwhelmed. The goal is not to be bursting with muscles, but to have enough strength to complete daily tasks and an extra reserve to allow more than the bare necessities. Strengthening may need to begin with using the weight of the FMS individual's own arm or leg as the weight. The starting point may be to move the arm as high as the shoulder 3-5 times and only gradually increase the height of the lift until it can move overhead without pain. Leg strengthening might begin with standing at the kitchen counter and rolling up and down from heels to toes or lifting a leg out to the side. Move through the exercises like floating on a cloud. Alternate movement with relax/release. Rest periods are important between each movement. Maintain a regular breathing rhythm without breath holding during the exercise. Avoid repetitively lowering arms and legs from a raised position – this is called an eccentric contraction – and is more fatiguing than moving them up and down.

Once exercise endurance has increased to ten repetitions of any one exercise without fatigue or residual soreness, weight or resistance can be used. Since commercial weights start at one pound it may be better to start with a 4-6 oz. can of tuna or mushrooms. Progress to 8 oz. of tomato paste, then 10 oz. of soup. Progress through the cupboard until a one pound weight is tolerated. If gripping a weight increases forearm pain, put dried beans or popcorn (unpopped, of course!) in a zip lock bag or in a knee high nylon and tie it around the wrist. It should slide on and off and allow the hand and forearm muscles to remain relaxed. Sometimes weights cause increased pain during and after exercise. This may be due to the resistance during the eccentric portion of the exercise, the resistance while returning to the rest position. Elastic bands or tubing is recommended as an alternative since there is no additional resistance during the eccentric portion of the exercise.

Large elastic bands or tubing come in a range of resistance from easy to difficult. The amount of resistance can be varied within one band by shortening it to make it harder or lengthening it to make it easier to pull against. A variety of exercises can be done with one band with a minimum of effort, whereas a series of weights are needed for different exercises. In FMS, elastic bands sometimes enable more exercise repetitions without soreness when compared to weights.

AEROBIC EXERCISE

Aerobic exercise is designed to deliver oxygen to tissues efficiently and improve heart and lung function. An individual with FMS needs to perform moderate aerobic exercise 5-6 times a week. Initially ask, "What can I do without increased pain?" Begin with "soft" non weight bearing exercises such as bicycling or water aerobics. Resting heart rate before starting exercise needs to be under 100 beats per minute, preferably 55-65 beats per minute. Use physiological quieting before aerobic exercise to lower heart rate and release tight muscle areas.

For inactive FMS individuals experiencing pain, start with a two minute warm up of gentle stretches with breathing, then perform three minutes of moderate exercise that increases heart rate towards the target heart rate. Then perform two minutes of warm down stretches with breathing release. Water exercises in warm water (85°F) at shoulder height enables more movement without pain.

For active FMS individuals exercising but experiencing pain, start with a 5-10 minute warm up of stretches, then progress to moderate exercise so there is not significant pain during or at the completion of the exercise. Insert rest cycles between shorter exercise cycles. For example, an individual may be used to running three miles daily feeling pain increase after two miles and being exhausted and painful for 4-6 hours after completion of the workout. The modified workout after warm up stretches would be running one mile, resting and/ or walking for five minutes, running for one mile, resting and/or walking for five minutes, then running for one mile, and cool down. If the individual is still sore and fatigued for 4-6 hours, decrease the work sets to one-half to three quarters of a mile each. End the exercise period with 5-10 minutes of cool down stretches. Doing the post exercise stretches and relaxation in a hot tub or under a hot shower is advisable to increase circulation that has decreased abnormally in the FMS individual's muscles.

Since FMS individuals' breathing patterns become erratic during exercise, it is important to be conscious of diaphragmatic breathing during aerobic exercise and rest cycles. Start with exercise that enables the maintenance of comfortable, rhythmical breathing. Some individuals will begin with walking a few blocks, a few lengths of a hallway or keeping time or dancing to one song on the radio. Aerobic activity utilizing equipment includes biking, using a tread-mill, cross country ski machine or steps.

Improvement in aerobic conditioning can be expected in 12-20 weeks, not in the six weeks expected aerobic progression with a non-FMS individual. The most important considerations are consistency of exercise and gradual increase in exercise tolerance. It is common to reach plateaus that last weeks or even a month or two. Don't give up. Maintain the exercise level that is comfortable.

When joining a group activity or joining a friend for tennis, golf, or bowling, the FMS individual may need to modify some of the movements or the pace to allow work within his/her limits. Start with fewer games or holes then gradually work up.

When starting with a new exercise or weight, do only 3-5 repetitions and see if there is any soreness the next day. Do not do a lot the first time even though there isn't any feeling of discomfort because the soreness may be delayed for several hours or even a day. If the same level of exercise is tolerated for three to four days without any negative effects then it is permissible to increase weight or repetitions, but only increase one of these at a time. Increase 1-2 repetitions at a time. Increase by a quarter to one half pound at a time. Give the 3-5 repetition prescription to any physical therapist that helps you.

POOL EXERCISES

Most exercises can be accomplished with less pain and faster progression if done in a warm pool. Aerobic exercise is also very effective in shoulder level warm water. The recommended target heart rate is approximately 20% less than recommended target heart rate for aerobic exercise on land. Aerobic endurance improves from 3-5 minutes for the acutely painful FMS individual to 45 minutes with 1-2 rest periods when the pain and fatigue has decreased. There should be no pain during pool exercise. The FMS individual should feel better at the end of the session even though there is a tired feeling. It is common for an individual to comment that it seems so easy in the pool. It is important not to overdo initially. Build up gradually. Always keep warm, using a hot tub or sauna and warm shower before and after the exercises. The pool temperature is best between 87-92° F to increase circulation and improve muscle relaxation. Being shoulder height in water eliminates 80% of gravity's pull on the body so movement can be the most efficient and pain-free.

WARM-UP STRETCHES
(DON'T FORGET TO BREATHE)
1. Neck – forward/back to neutral
   – side bend
   – rotation
2. Shoulders – hand to opposite shoulder
3. Wrist – forward/back, circles each direction, turn palms up/down
4. Leg/hip – hamstring stretch, Achilles stretch, hip rotator stretch, adductors stretch

EXERCISES IN STANDING
I. Standing arm exercises while marching
   A. Arms forward/backward
   B. Hand circles
   C. Hands to opposite shoulders
   D. Arms forward & back – hand by face height
   E. One hand on abdomen, one hand on low back, then reverse
   F. Elbows to shoulder height, then down
   G. Bend elbows, push down

II. Standing leg exercises
   A. Marching
   B. Weight shift right, to left, feet apart
   C. Rock forward (elbows back), rock back (arms forward)
   D. Leg out to side

    E. Leg back & forward

    F. Leg circles

III. Arm and leg exercises

    A. Hand to opposite knee

    B. Hand toward opposite foot

    C. Hand to inside heel

    D. Hand to outside heel

    E. Hands to right, legs to left – twist, then reverse

IV. Water walking – forward, backward, side crossovers

CHAPTER 12

WHAT CAN I DO TO STAY EMOTIONALLY HEALTHY?

Ellen S. Silverglat, M.S.W
Janet A. Hulme, P.T.

Having an illness lets us know that an individual is not invulnerable to the problems that others suffer. People like to believe that illness and accidents happen to others. Sometimes an FMS individual resorts to superstition to reassure him/herself. As a part of an audience at a presentation where the odds of getting a disease or having an accident are stated, think about the fact that people all through the group are counting friends and family who have already had the problem and then giving a sigh of relief as if some quota had been met that spared them. It is easy to spot unrealistic perceptions of invulnerability or even immortality among adolescents. Adults are less obvious but it lingers on in many people. To admit that you can develop a medical problem is to admit lack of control and the absence of guarantees in our lives. Often people ask, "Why has this happened to me?" which almost sounds like others deserve the problem. Acknowledging that unwanted changes can happen may affect our self image if it was believed previously that illness equals weakness or lack of sufficient vigilance on our part to stay well. Just as an individual is not wholly defined by his/her work, his lineage, his physical attributes or any other single factor, he/she is not defined by this state of health. Part of the work of staying emotionally healthy is remembering how complex each individual is. Reduced strength in some areas doesn't cancel an individual's personality. Modification of how an individual performs daily activities doesn't cancel wit, sense of humor or other good or bad traits.

An individual's opinions of him/herself may be based on inaccurate information and lead to harsh self appraisal. Information about what each individual must deal with can alleviate a lot of self blame, feelings of persecution or disappointment resulting from unrealistic expectations. Although the fund of information on fibromyalgia may be incomplete, it is a healthy thing to seek reliable information. Being well informed is part of being a responsible person. The unknown is often worse than reality and fear of the unknown leads to increased anxiety and poor coping. Watch out for myths such as "all illnesses are acute, lab tests and x-ray can diagnose everything, there are cures for almost everything, strength of will can overcome any disease" or the devastating thought that "chronic illness means a meaningful life is ended." Positive thoughts alone may not be a cure but they can greatly enhance coping. Negative thoughts can make any illness worse and immobilize coping abilities.

What does it mean that an FMS individual has a need to see one or more health care professionals? It doesn't mean he/she must or should relinquish all decision making to these people. Sometimes it is hard to remember that the individual is a very important part of his/her care. Many times an FMS individual is the only one in the room who isn't wearing "real clothes." Everyone else may be wearing street clothes or even uniforms while he/she wears a gown. The other people are active, and at times being a "patient" requires being passive. The care givers give instructions, medicines, and therapy to the "patient." All of the above might imply that the patient does nothing important and that is inaccurate and demoralizing. Being a "patient" is only one of numerous roles and not an entire identity. Remember that when the doctor goes to the dentist he or she has that role. In the clinical setting, the FMS individual's job is to participate and become an active member of the team. When the "patient" clothing is shed, the individual's job is to go about the business of leading as full a life as possible. Being an active, involved and key member of the treatment plan is emotionally rewarding.

While doing so, it is important to keep in mind one critical distinction. Being a responsible "patient" and participating actively in self care does not mean that the FMS individual is to blame for having the illness in the first place. An FMS individual would never think such a cruel thing about someone with cancer or arthritis, so a reminder of "I didn't cause this" is important.

Anger is a common emotion when dealing with fibromyalgia. Feeling angry for a long time without discovering a way to safely express it or even acknowledge it is a burden. It is easier to talk about anger if there is a villain to target. When illness happens, anger is directed in many directions because usually there is no one responsible to direct it at. Many people have the idea that feeling angry is a bad thing. An individual can't help feeling an emotion, and experiencing it isn't the problem. The big problem is what is done with the feeling. Taking anger out on others is a harmful way to let the feelings out. Others are not responsible for what has occurred in the FMS individual's life.

Companionship and friendship of friends and family is needed, and widespread resentment makes it difficult for these people to be close. Sometimes the worst outbursts of frustration and anger are inflicted on those who care for an FMS individual the most and are closest to him/her. They are the safest and most likely to still show love after the outburst. They are easily available targets for frustrated feelings and anger.

A sense of unfairness and fear of being dependent are often part of that anger. The fear of increased dependence causing those closest to an FMS individual to pull away is really frightening. Sadly, this fear can lead to behavior that makes it much more likely that the worst fears will be realized.

Anger turned inward is also not the answer. Anger turned inward often results in depression. Why is it so hard to handle this emotion with a chronic illness? Perhaps an individual confuses acceptance of the situation with liking what has happened. The angry feeling may be a way to let him/herself and the rest of the world know that this is really awful and it should go away. Accepting facts doesn't mean liking them or choosing the situation. Acceptance means working with reality and choosing to have more of life rather than less.

This brings back the subject of control. Genuine control is working with what an FMS individual has and not falling prey to the superman or victim role. Control helps perspective. Not only the person with fibromyalgia has bad and good days, so does everyone else. Before a person gets a diagnosis they can accept ups and downs in life as a matter of course, why not after? Having a bad spell is not justification for writing off the future. Plan for the future based on what can be done, not on what was possible in the past or on what should be done, or on what others do. Do not confuse this information with some glib slogan (make

93

lemonade out of lemons). This is an attempt to overcome the real danger of giving up and settling for less than is deserved.

Finding ways to use anger to motivate rather than block action, ways to appropriately ask for help and to say "no thank you" to offers of help, and ways to exercise control in life are some of the things to be learned. There are times when things aren't going well and the FMS individual feels sad and angry but be aware that those who care the most may feel inadequate or overwhelmed by the situation. An objective person who understands feelings but is not personally involved in the FMS individual's life is a safer person to talk with and is someone who can make observations that loved ones don't see or are afraid to mention.

If you do not have a pet, think seriously about getting one. Studies have shown that companion animals are beneficial to the physical and mental health of human beings. Walking a dog is the one form of exercise some individuals can do. It doesn't require club membership or a schedule with a friend to do it. There are less energetic interactions too . . . rolling a ball or dangling a ribbon for a cat. Always there is the company and affection of a living being happy for our companionship whether we are in a bad or good mood. If pets aren't allowed in your home or apartment, ask friends to share their animals or visit the humane society.

Judy, who has had fibromyalgia for six years, describes her priorities for staying emotionally healthy stating:

"1. Learn to say 'No' to things you don't want to do.
2. Value your time and give some to yourself each day.
3. Take time to exercise daily 20-30 minutes.
4. Walk away from stressful situations that are not yours.
5. Practice physiological quieting and meditation daily."

CHAPTER 13

WHAT CAN I DO
TO BE ACTIVE AT HOME?

Joyce Dougan, P.T.
Janet A. Hulme, P. T.

The important tasks necessary for the function of a daily household can be overwhelming to someone who is in pain and feels fatigue. Household jobs are repetitive by nature so having a plan or schedule that prioritizes the FMS individual's comfort as equal importance to the day's endeavors is essential. Initially, list the week's jobs and distribute them over the seven days. Next, decide who will do each job, delegating to family members and hired help some of the tasks that cause the most pain and fatigue. Now, break up each task into smaller units and spread the units out through that day. For example, take rests between each room when vacuuming. Additionally, another job's sub task (chopping vegetables for dinner) can be done after the rest period and before the vacuuming is done again. Varying the tasks varies the muscles used and the movement patterns performed by the same muscles which decreases the possibility of pain and fatigue.

Spring house cleaning tasks should be hired out or spread

throughout the year and involve the whole family. Yard work and gardening need to be low maintenance. Care free landscaping with evergreens, rocks and chips can be colorful with little care. Plastic under flower and vegetable gardens minimizes weeding. Use of raised beds saves strain on knees and back muscles. Pots of flowers or even vegetables can be placed in or out of the house and need minimal care.

In the kitchen, organization of space and design can assist in comfortable meal preparation. Place frequently used objects within easy reach so there is minimal reaching overhead or a need to stoop to lift something. Pots and pans which are the heaviest need to be at the same level as the stove. Use a step stool to reach the cupboards that are overhead and sit on it to reach into the lowest cupboards. Whenever possible use light weight pots, pans, and dishes. Do food preparation seated at a table using an office chair with wheels rather than standing at the sink or counter. In the sink, raise the washing surface by placing a dish pan on top of four cups or plastic containers. At the counter use a thick cutting board or place equipment on 4x4s to elevate the work surface so there is minimal bending forward when working.

Planning meals a week at a time lets others help with grocery shopping on their days off. Carrying heavy bags to and from the car is a task where help is often needed. Cooking meals using crock pots or making large portions of casseroles, lasagne or spaghetti can provide two days' meals instead of one. Planning one takeout meal or a frozen meal once a week gives the flexibility to not cook when a day has been particularly stressful. Buying children's cookbooks encourages them to cook a meal.

Laundry is a task that can be aggravating to fibromyalgia symptoms unless pacing and simplification strategies are used. Wash one load a day instead of three or four a day. Let each family member do their own laundry when they are old enough to use the washing machine (9-10 years old). At least have each family member sort their dirty clothes before someone washes and dries them, then they can pick up the clean clothes, fold and return them to their closets. Hire out ironing and buy wash and wear clothes. Underwear and sheets don't need ironing. Just fold underwear and lay sheets on the bed after drying. Have a basket of towels and wash-cloths unfolded that family members can use as they are needed. Those clothes that need folding can be folded on a counter top or while sitting at a table.

Bathroom cleaning can be simplified too. Clean and wipe down the tub after the shower or bath but while still in it. Use a long handled scrubber for reaching in the shower or tub to clean them. Wipe off the sink and toilet every other day as they are used. Use mild cleaning agents since some individuals are hypersensitive to chemicals.

Bill paying and letter writing are more comfortable using a fine felt tipped pen on a slanted writing surface. When a computer keyboard is used, rest it on a pillow or lap board at elbow height in the lap. If the telephone is used much, a headset or speaker phone rather than manually holding the phone or securing the phone between the head and shoulder helps keep the FMS individual's neck and jaw from hurting.

Shopping can be an exhausting event or a pleasurable experience depending on the planning that precedes the event. If walking and driving are problems, use mail order to purchase clothes, kitchen equipment, gifts, even shoes. Check on delivery services available in your area. Often they will do your shopping for you if you provide the list. Comparison shop by phone to find the best buys before making up a list. When planning to go out to shop, plan short trips and organize a list of items for different locations. Then go to one or two locations a day. Get a handicapped parking sticker from the local city/county offices. Use the wheelchairs or electric scooters available in stores. Say "yes" to offers of help in carrying shopping bags to the car.

WHAT CAN I DO TO TRAVEL COMFORTABLY?

Traveling creates new challenges for the individual with FMS. The physical act of driving can take the pleasure out of traveling for someone with FMS. Taxis, buses, trains and planes can be used for travel without having to do the physical act of driving. Baggage assistance is usually available and should be utilized. Check all luggage and arrange door to door shuttle service to the destination before leaving home. When driving or riding in a car, well fitting back and arm supports are important. Get out, stretch and walk around frequently, usually at least every hour. For long trips, break up each day with longer rest periods by reclining in the back seat, visiting tourist sites while taking short walks, or having a picnic. Complete driving early in the day and stay where there is a hot tub and/or pool to use. When staying over night away from home, have the pillow and eggcrate mattress from home. Remember to take sleep aids like ear plugs or a white noise machine. After arrival at the destination, pace the planned activities. Staying in one place and taking short side trips often works well. Keeping regular dietary habits and a medication schedule are important for an enjoyable vacation.

CHAPTER 14

WHAT CAN I DO TO SUCCESSFULLY WORK?

Joyce Dougan, P.T.
Ellen S. Silverglat, M.S.W.
Janet A. Hulme, P.T.

No examination of living with fibromyalgia is complete without looking at work. It is important to change the work environment because little things at work can result in enormous suffering later on. People working 40 hours per week spend approximately one third of the day on the job. It is likely that no other activity, including being with family and recreation, takes up such large blocks of time. Only the number of hours slept may approach the amount one works. Work is not only a big factor because of the amount of time spent at professions and employment, it is significant because of the reasons an individual works. In addition to providing financially for themselves and their dependents, an individual acquires part of their sense of identity from his/her work. In the best circumstances an FMS individual derives a sense of satisfaction from work that goes beyond the monetary compensation. The workplace is also an opportunity for socializing. Being able to continue to do one's work competently is of great concern to anyone with a chronic illness.

When an individual is concerned about being able to handle all of his/her duties there is often the urge to take a marathon approach to the job. This might include skipping breaks or lunch hours in order to spend as much time as possible "being productive." The same rationale may encourage overtime, not occasionally but routinely. This approach does not accomplish the desired goal, but it does affect the individual negatively. Quantity and quality of work actually decreases and the worker becomes less efficient. Typically it is common for the overworking individual to become more irritable, more fatigued and restless, and less positive about the work or his/her abilities. Anxiety about job performance can actually exacerbate the very symptoms one worries about interfering with performance.

There are approaches to doing one's job that can diminish fears and lessen tension. Take coffee and lunch breaks on schedule. Use half of the fifteen minute break to loosen muscles, get fresh air, or chat about something not work related. At lunch time instead of eating at the desk or in the room, eat outside and take a walk after eating. Even running errands is probably better than feeling chained to the desk. If there isn't anyone to talk with, bring a book and read a chapter. Try using visualization techniques between tasks or on breaks. Use exercises the therapist outlined for breathing and relaxing specific muscles.

Interpersonal relationships are a benefit of working but they can also be a stressor. Not all coworkers, peers and supervisors get along well. Personal problems, personality traits, and illness can affect how one relates to others. Spending a number of hours around someone difficult can be uncomfortable, but keeping the situation in perspective can help. Keep in mind that this person's primary role in your life is that of fellow employee, not friend. If working with a particular person is too stressful, talk to the personnel office or to the appropriate supervisor. It may be that at times the FMS individual blames illness for bad days when other factors that are hard to confront are a big part of the cause. Don't assume negative feelings probably are due to illness or medication. Having fibromyalgia or any other disease does not make someone exempt from everyday stressors.

What about those days when fibromyalgia flares up? Sometimes it is necessary to take sick days or time off for appointments. Even if the employer doesn't care about individual employee's health problems, it is usually a wise move to briefly explain the facts of the necessary treatment. Brief knowledge of the FMS individual's situation may make time for medical appointments less of an issue for co-workers and supervisors. Unless working with a good friend who will keep confidences, it is advisable not to discuss discomforts in great detail. Extensive descriptions of medical problems can get in the way of being viewed and treated as a peer. Remember everyone comes to the work place with some unique situation and hearing a lot about any one problem gets old.

Coming home from work is a time of transition, an adjustment from work to home. It is a good idea to allow a 30-60 minute period of time to make that transition. Some people read the mail, watch the news, change clothes, take a walk, or even grab a quick catnap. Ask family members to postpone non emergencies for the first 20 minutes to half hour so there is time to switch gears. This is a chance to let go of physical and mental stress from work and approach the role at home without that burden. If rest or a nap is needed after work, make a schedule that allows that routinely. The same rule applies to exercise or any other health maintenance routine. To help get the most out of the "quiet time" during the transition from work to home, have the evening meal prepared ahead of time. Solutions can be a crock pot or oven meal, a quick microwave meal or a takeout meal.

In the workplace there are many modifications to equipment, dress, and movement patterns that make the job easier and more efficient. Change positions frequently. For some individuals with FMS it will be necessary to change as often as every 15 minutes while for others every 30 minutes will be adequate. After sitting for a period of time, stand up and stretch or walk a short distance. After a time of standing, sit or walk for a short period. This change uses different muscle groups and decreases fatigue and pain.

For a standing job it is important to wear good supportive shoes. A building is only as good as its foundation and feet are the body's foundation. The work surface height is important in a standing job to protect the back. A general guideline is to have the surface approximately elbow height. Lifts can be put under table legs or legs can be cut off. A very simple and cost effective piece of equipment to increase standing tolerance is a rubberized floor mat. They are available through catalogues or in hardware or restaurant supply stores.

If the primary work position is sitting, it is important to have a well fitted chair that offers good support for back and hips. The chair should allow the feet to be flat on the floor, the seat should be of adequate width to support the buttocks and thighs and deep enough so the seat ends about three inches from the back of the knee. The chair back should provide low back support to keep weight directly over ischial tuberosities or "butt bones." The shoulders and head will then more easily balance over the hips with less muscular effort.

If work is performed while seated at a desk, the height of the desk and the position of the equipment on it are important considerations. The desk top should generally be at elbow height when sitting with back supported. If the desk is too high and requires shoulders and arms to be elevated all day there will be increased discomfort and decreased productivity. If it isn't feasible to lower a desk the chair can be adjusted to a higher level with a foot rest added to keep the feet supported. When working on a computer the keyboard can often be put on a pullout shelf below the desktop to obtain the correct height.

Equipment location on a desk is important for the individual with FMS. Equipment used most often should be closest to the individual. This might mean rearranging the phone, calculator, rolodex, or computer. If the calculator is used a lot during the day, move it to midline so the individual's elbow can be at his/her side or resting on the desk when using the keyboard. Always have the computer monitor in midline at eye level 36 inches or one full arm's length away from your face. Position the keyboard close to the body and at approximately elbow height.

Some new equipment can decrease mechanical stresses on the job. A headset is essential if there is much phone work. Arm and wrist supports can be essential to improved production with less pain. A document holder can keep the head and neck comfortable when transposing data from documents to the computer.

The physical work environment – temperature, noise, lighting, and vibration – affects how the FMS individual feels and his/her productivity. These stressors can increase pain, stiffness and fatigue. If temperature is a problem, experiment with layering clothing and wearing silk turtlenecks, even in summer. If an air conditioning vent is positioned directly over the work area, check to see if it can be closed or angled differently or have a deflector placed on the vent. If noise is excessive, try ear plugs or use a headset with quiet music or nature sounds. Lighting can be angled differently or additional lighting can be added. Full spectrum overhead lights are more expensive but the cost is offset by the improved health and productivity of the employees. Rubber mats to stand on can absorb vibration. They can be put under desk and chair legs to decrease vibration from the environment to work surfaces.

In addition to having a good physical work setting, there is also the need to use the body efficiently. Learn to use only the muscles required for a task and keep the others relaxed. Use the necessary muscles as if they are floating through the task. Biofeedback can help achieve efficient muscle use first in the clinic and then at the job site.

Using good body mechanics during lifting, carrying, reaching, pushing and pulling is essential for comfort and efficiency. When lifting, it is recommended that feet be at least shoulder width apart and one slightly ahead of the other to provide a firm base of support. Bend knees, not the back, to get close to the item and lift while keeping the object close to the body. Keep the head up and exhale while lifting to help stabilize the back. When moving an item from one level to another (a laundry basket from floor to table) turn by walking rather than pivoting and twisting at the waist. Carrying with two hands is most effectively done with the weight held at waist level. When carrying an item at chest height the hips tend to lean backwards to help maintain the individual's balance. This increases back strain. When carrying something in one hand at the side, like a 12 pack of pop, try to put something of comparable weight in the other hand for equal balance. When pushing an item, place one foot in front of the other so there is weight shift from the back foot to the front foot to initiate movement. Have the item to be pushed as directly in front of the body as possible to avoid twisting.

At times it is necessary to change jobs, decrease the hours you work or not work at all for a period of time because of fibromyalgia symptoms. The physician, physical or occupational therapist, or vocational rehabilitation specialist can assist in analyzing the situation. Part time work may be an option, a change in job description, or a new job that better fits the individual's needs are options to consider. Sometimes self employment is the best choice for the FMS individual since he/she can work at his/her own pace and accept contracts that are doable. Retraining, education for a new occupation, and career counseling are all options to consider when the present job is not the best alternative.

The Americans with Disability Act (ADA) describes that a qualified individual with a disability who can perform the essential functions of his/her job cannot be discriminated against. The employer is required to make reasonable accommodations for the worker unless it would impose undue hardship.

CHAPTER 15

WHAT CAN I DO TO
HAVE FUN AND PLAY?

Joyce Dougan, P.T.
Ellen S. Silverglat, M.S.W.
Janet A. Hulme, P.T.

Fun and play are part of every individual's balanced life-style. The individual with fibromyalgia has the need for fun and play as much or more than anyone else. Many times when asked "What do you do for fun?" the FMS individual responds "I work" or "I don't have time for fun and play." The idea that work is what is really important and play is a sideline for the lazy can be replaced with the idea that there needs to be a balance of work, play, and rest to be healthy. Some FMS individuals describe waiting to play until the pain is gone or until a new medicine is found to cure them before they play. Instead the FMS individual must look for the new medicine but continue to have balance in everyday life through fun and play. The thought that play and leisure is a luxury of the past and no longer a possibility with FMS can be replaced with the idea that play and leisure are a necessity, not a luxury. Sometimes FMS individuals respond "I might injure myself or make things worse; I'm too fragile now." The replacement thought is "I can learn to play safely."

Sometimes the fear of failure gets in the way of fun and play. The FMS individual thinks, "I must be able to play the way I did before." The replacement thought is, "There is more than one way to enjoy myself and the search for the new ways can be fun." Some FMS individuals say "Competition is the key, without it there is no point in a recreational activity. Those other activities are for wimps." The replacement thought pattern can be, "Really? Wouldn't something be better than nothing?" The thought that "I can't learn a new activity now that I have this problem" sometimes puts a roadblock up to fun and play. The question to ask is "Have I tried? What do I have to lose ?"

The individual with FMS must focus on what he/she can realistically do. Instead of the thought, "I can't run 5 miles a day so I won't do anything" say, "I can go for walks with friends along the river." Instead of the thought, "I'll swim 3000 yards even if I can't get out of bed tomorrow," say, "I'll do water aerobics for 30 minutes in a warm pool." The focus is on what the individual can do in comfort and without extreme fatigue while having fun and "playing."

Redefining fun and play is a gradual process. The exercise to "Think of what you did as a child, then as an adolescent for fun and play. What activities that you did then might be fun now?" is often helpful in coming up with 'new ideas' for fun and play. As a child you painted pictures and admired them. By suspending judgement and just "doing," the joy of noncompetitive fun returns.

Another question to ask is, "What are the fun and play activities I've always thought I might try? How can I modify them so I can enjoy the new event and feel OK the next day?" There is never a better time to find out how to do something new. Maybe it's archery or horseback riding that interests you. Plan to take lessons from a professional and adjust the time spent to your energy and pain level. If the roadblock is "I might get too tired or sore and have to go slow or even stop for awhile" discuss this with the instructor and plan rest periods ahead of time. Developing new hobbies can add variety to leisure time. New crafts, bird watching, flower arranging, photography, collecting old toy trucks at garage sales, are all possibilities. Using a computer to make new friends and to play computer games can be a whole new world. Dream about what might be interesting and fun. Then try it!

Often the question of, "How do I go on excursions with friends when I know I won't be able to keep up with them?" comes up. The solution may be to plan parallel play with meeting places along the way for conversation and meals. For example, on a cross-country ski excursion with friends, the FMS individual may go at his/her pace with frequent rests while the others are on a more difficult trail at a faster pace but there is a planned meeting time and place for lunch to compare notes and enjoy the company. When vacations are planned, the FMS individual may plan to fly to the destination while others drive.

In all leisure and play, plan ahead to make the event pleasant. Obtain a handicapped parking permit and find out where the parking area is. Take a back cushion or special chair when the event requires sitting. Sit at the end of the aisle so you can get up and move around. Use a stadium seat if the event's seating is on bleachers. Take a change of clothes or wear layers for the possibility of weather and temperature changes. Take healthy snacks and water.

Entertaining at home means preparing food several days ahead of time or having meals catered. Housecleaning can also be done ahead and delegated to family members or hired out. The day before the event it is important to plan rest periods interspersed in the day's work. During the event having a quiet place to spend five minutes resting can help make the event pleasant for you as well as the guests.

Creating a positive outlook about leisure activities means building a thought framework to support fun. Expecting to enjoy yourself whether alone or in the company of others is a part of fun and leisure. Changing negative thoughts to positive "I can try" thoughts is essential. Avoiding tunnel vision about what is a fun activity and enjoying many aspects of any activity lets fun come into everyday life. Everyone benefits from enjoying the process, the path, not just the end result of leisure and fun activities.

Rest beforehand, rest along the way, learn pacing with the idea of not hurting the next day. Discuss with companions and family the "comfort zone" of activity. Build up gradually in endurance over a 2-3 month period. Know that fun and play are their own reward. Fun and play are as important to schedule as work and rest.

CHAPTER 16

WHAT CAN MY FAMILY DO TO HELP?

Ellen S. Silverglat, M.S.W.
Janet A. Hulme, P.T.

Families become involved in the FMS individual's care, attitude, and goals. Family members need to become educated about fibromyalgia. It isn't simple to explain, but it is worth the effort. Explain to family members that, "yes, it is real, no there is no cure for it, and yes I can deal with it. I wish it would go away too, but it won't."

Let family members know there will be bad days and good days. "I will be as active as is possible and as is good for me." A mother will explain, "some days you may have to iron your own shirt or make your own lunch."

Understand that a "bad mood" may be a part of fibromyalgia or it may just be a bad mood. This illness doesn't explain everything about the individual. "The same stuff that irritated me before bothers me now. The same things that delighted me before please me now."

Relax, a person with fibromyalgia won't break. "I am not an invalid. I am not dying. Some days I am more incapacitated than others, some days I need more attention than others. You can help by doing more for yourself but I am still your wife, mother, or daughter."

Fibromyalgia is an illness, not an excuse. "None of us should use it to explain away things. All of us need to be honest."

The symptoms of fibromyalgia are real – headaches, back pain, gut pain, fatigue, confusion – all are real, they come and go. "Please don't pretend my symptoms don't exist, don't ridicule me or put me down when I tell you how I feel. Just say 'I hear you, it's not your fault.'"

Families learn that doing less may mean being able to do more in the case of someone with fibromyalgia. Daily schedules let the family know what activity limits there are and when there are rest times scheduled. Then there is not the need for a family member to ask "Are you sure you want to do this?" or "Do you feel so bad you need to take a break?"

Family members need reassurance that you are in control. "I don't need a keeper. I'm happy being quiet sometimes. I'm responsible for seeing to my own health care. I'll ask for help when I need it."

Half a loaf is better than none in the case of fibromyalgia. "I can feel sorry for myself if I need to, but don't encourage it. I'll take advantage of opportunities to live my life to the fullest. Thank you for your support."

Care but please don't hover or try to disprove how the individual with FMS feels or believes. "If I need to hibernate, don't rebut me. If you read an article in a magazine that says fibromyalgia is due to poor spiritual life, don't be eager to tell me. If your best friend's aunt who has fibromyalgia dropped dead . . . or ate a diet of dandelions and never ached again . . . or joined a cult to deal with fibromyalgia, please understand that I may be disinclined to do the same."

Illnesses of unknown cause invite unproved remedies. Don't undermine the treatments that are trusted and comfortable for the individual with fibromyalgia.

"When I whine, just say you are sorry it's a bad day and you hope things will improve. They will."

"Let me care for you when you aren't feeling well. It's important to be able to give back."

RESOURCES

The American Fibromyalgia Syndrome Association
P.O. Box 9699
Bakersfield, CA 93389

The Fibromyalgia Network Newsletter
P.O. Box 31750
Tucson, AZ 85751

Phoenix Seminars
P.O. Box 8231
Missoula, MT 59807
1-800-549-8371

Arthritis Foundation
P.O. Box 19000
Atlanta, GA 30326

Phoenix Publishing Catalogue
P.O. Box 8231
Missoula, MT 59807
1-800-549-8371
    Self care items, books, and tapes

Suggested Readings

Sick and Tired of Feeling Sick and Tired – Living with Invisible Chronic Illness, Paul Donoghue, Ph.D. and Mary E. Siegel, Ph.D., New York: W.W. Norton & Company.

When Muscle Pain Won't Go Away, Gayle Backstrom, Taylor Publishing, Dallas, TX, 1992.

Fibromyalgia, Managing the Pain, Mark Pellegrino, M.D., Anadem Publishing, Columbus, Ohio, 1993.

Myofascial Pain and Fibromyalgia, Edward S. Rachlin, Mosby Publishing, Boston, 1994.

Musculoskeletal Pain, Myofascial Pain Syndrome, and the Fibromyalgia Syndrome, Soren Jacobsen, Bente Danneskiold-Samsoe, Birger Lund, Haworth Medical Press, New York, 1993.

Soft and Easy Exercise, M. Bennett, J. Palmquist. Fitness is My Business, Helena, MT 1997.

Managing Fibromyalgia: A Six Week Course on Self Care, B. Penner, Capital P.T., Helena MT, 1997.

The Honest Herbal, Varro Tyler, Haworth Medical Press, 1993.

Fibromyalgia & Chronic Myofascial Pain Syndrome – A Survival Manual, Devin Starlanyl, Mary Ellen Copeland, Oakland CA., New Harbinger Publishing, 1996.

Computer Networks

Ability OnLine
1919 Alness St.
North York ON M3J2J1
Modem: 416-650-5411
Internet e-mail: infor@ablelink.org

Videotapes /Audiotapes

Physiological Quieting Audiotape
Phoenix Publishing
P.O. Box 8231
Missoula, MT 59807
1-800-549-8371

Fibromyalgia: Face to Face
Fibromyalgia Association
250 Bloor St. E., Suite 905
Toronto, Ontario M4W 3P2 Canada

Fitness Is My Business
628 Mound
Helena, MT 59601

Fibromyalgia Exercise Video
Oakville-Trafalgar Memorial Hospital
327 Reynolds Street
Oakville, Ontario L61 3L7 Canada

NOTES:

ORDER FORM

I would like to order additional copies of
Fibromyalgia, A Handbook for Self Care and Treatment

1-9 Copies $14.95 ea.   10 or more copies $10.95 ea.

No. of copies_____   x **$14.95** = _____

No. of copies_____   x **$10.95** = _____

Shipping & Handling (1st copy)   = **$3.00**

Each additional copy **$.50**   = _____

Total Cost of Order $ _____

Please send check or money order to:

Phoenix Publishing Co.
P.O. Box 8231
Missoula, MT 59807
1-800-549-8371

Name_____

Address _____

City_____State____Zip _____

Telephone (_____) _____

117